THE CHOLESTEROL COUNTER

ANNETTE NATOW, Ph.D., R.D., and JO-ANN HESLIN, M.A., R.D., are the authors of seven books on nutrition, including *The Pocket Encyclopedia of Nutrition, No-Nonsense Nutrition for Kids* and *Megadoses: Vitamins as Drugs* (all available from Pocket Books). They are faculty members of Adelphi University and previously taught at Downstate Medical Center and New York University. They have held editorial positions at the *Journal of Nutrition for the Elderly, American Baby* and *Prevention* magazines, and are regular contributors to *Redbook,* health magazines and journals.

Books by Annette Natow and Jo-Ann Heslin

The Cholesterol Counter
Megadoses
No-Nonsense Nutrition for Kids
The Pocket Encyclopedia of Nutrition

Published by POCKET BOOKS

Most Pocket Books are available at special quantity discounts for bulk purchases for sales promotions, premiums or fund raising. Special books or book excerpts can also be created to fit specific needs.

For details write the office of the Vice President of Special Markets, Pocket Books, 1230 Avenue of the Americas, New York, New York 10020.

THE CHOLESTEROL COUNTER

Annette B. Natow, Ph.D., R.D.
Jo-Ann Heslin, M.A., R.D.

Another *Original* publication of POCKET BOOKS

POCKET BOOKS, a division of Simon & Schuster, Inc.
1230 Avenue of the Americas, New York, N.Y. 10020

Copyright © 1988 by Annette B. Natow and Jo-Ann Heslin

ISBN: 0-671-68274-1

First Pocket Books printing April 1988

10 9 8 7 6 5 4 3 2 1

POCKET and colophon are trademarks of
Simon & Schuster, Inc.

Cover design by Mike Stromberg

Printed in the U.S.A.

To our families, who support us through every project:
Harry, Allen, Irene, Sarah, Laura, Marty, George, Steven,
Joseph, Kristen and Karen

ACKNOWLEDGMENTS

Without the tireless cooperation of Steven and Laura, *Cholesterol Counter* would never have been completed. A special thanks to Abe and Lillie Lefkowitz who were there when we really needed them.

Our thanks also go to all the food manufacturers who graciously shared their data.

AUTHORS' NOTE

Values in this counter have been obtained from the U.S. Department of Agriculture, Bowes and Church's *Food Values of Portions Commonly Used* (Philadelphia, PA: J.B. Lippincott Co., 1985), *Nutrients in Foods* (Cambridge, MA: Nutrition Guild, 1983) and information from food labels, manufacturers and processors. The values are based on research conducted prior to 1988. Manufacturer's ingredients are subject to change, so current values may vary from those listed in the book.

"If only half a dozen foods were available, the matter would be quickly settled."

MARY SWARTZ ROSE, PH.D.
Feeding the Family
The MacMillan Company
1919

CONTENTS

WHAT IS CHOLESTEROL?

High cholesterol is a major risk factor for heart disease.
High cholesterol is a major risk factor for stroke.
High cholesterol increases your risk of colon and rectal cancer.
High cholesterol plus high blood pressure may cause hearing loss.
High cholesterol, fat-rich diets may cause gallstones.

Did you know that every year more than half a million Americans die from coronary heart disease—heart attack and stroke? That's more than the number of people who die from all forms of cancer! Heart attack and stroke disable even more people than they kill. Coronary heart disease is a disease not only of the old. One out of five men has a heart attack before he is fifty. Often, the heart attack or stroke that causes death or disability is the first sign you get that something is wrong.

Research shows that high cholesterol levels are one of the most important risk factors for heart disease. Lowering your cholesterol lowers your risk.

What is cholesterol?

Cholesterol is a white, waxy, fatlike substance that is part of every cell in your body. Cholesterol is important to body function. Hormones, nerve coverings, vitamin D, bile (used for digestion), and the fat that keeps your skin soft (sebum) are all made from cholesterol. Cholesterol makes up a major part of your brain. Cholesterol is needed by the body but when the blood level of cholesterol in your blood gets too high, it's not healthy. Some of that extra cholesterol can be deposited on the artery wall, narrowing it and interfering with normal blood flow.

Where does cholesterol come from?

We get some cholesterol every time we eat any animal foods. Meat, poultry, fish, eggs, milk, yogurt, cheese and butter are all animal foods and contain cholesterol. Egg yolk is a major source of cholesterol. An average yolk contains about 250 milligrams. The egg white does not have any cholesterol. Caviar and organ meats like liver, heart and brains are very high in cholesterol.

There is no cholesterol in any food that grows in the ground. Vegetable oils, peanut butter, vegetables, fruits, cereals and grains contain *no* cholesterol.

Cholesterol is also made in the body. In fact most people make three times as much cholesterol as they get in the food they eat.

How do I know if my blood cholesterol is too high?

A blood test done after you have not eaten for twelve hours can tell you your blood cholesterol level. Below are average blood cholesterol levels of Americans but they are not the most healthy levels.

AVERAGE BLOOD CHOLESTEROL LEVELS*

AGE	MALES	FEMALES
20–29	175	165
30–39	195	180
40–49	210	200
50–59	215	225
60–69	215	230
70 +	205	230

*Adapted from "American Heart Association Special Report: Recommendation for the Treatment of Hyperlipidemia: A Joint Statement of the Nutrition Committee and the Council on Arteriosclerosis of the American Heart Association," *Circulation*, 69(1984):433a.

For adults, a cholesterol level over 200 milligrams is considered too high. If your cholesterol is above 200 milligrams your risk for heart disease and other problems is increased.

CHOLESTEROL VALUES THAT PLACE YOU AT RISK*

AGE	MODERATE RISK	HIGH RISK
20–29	200–220	over 220
30–39	220–240	over 240
40 +	240–260	over 260

**"Lowering Blood Cholesterol to Prevent Heart Disease: Consensus Conference," *Journal of the American Medical Association*, 253(1985):2080.

If my cholesterol is higher than 200, what should I do?

In late 1987 the federal government along with over twenty health organizations, issued guidelines to help identify and treat people whose blood cholesterol levels are too high. *This will affect one in four Americans.*

People with desirable cholesterol levels of under 200 milligrams were advised only to recheck the level every 5 years.

People with levels above 200 milligrams are advised to go on a cholesterol lowering diet that is low in cholesterol, fats and saturated fats.

Many foods are high in all three—cholesterol, fats and saturated fats. By lowering your intake of high cholesterol foods, you reduce your intake of other fats as well and lower your risk for heart disease.

For each 1 percent decrease in blood cholesterol level, you reduce your risk of heart disease by 2 percent. Even the smallest change is to your benefit.

In the government guidelines for lowering cholesterol, the Step I diet for those whose cholesterol levels are 200 to 239 milligrams recommends eating less than 300 milligrams of cholesterol a day. Those people whose cholesterol levels are 240 milligrams and over are advised to restrict their cholesterol intake to less than 200 milligrams per day.

GUIDELINES FOR CHOLESTEROL INTAKE*

CHOLESTEROL LEVEL IN THE BLOOD	MG OF CHOLESTEROL YOU CAN EAT EACH DAY
200 to 239 mg	less than 300 mg a day
240 mg and over	less than 200 mg a day

*Adapted from material provided by National Cholesterol Education Program, National Heart, Lung and Blood Institute, National Institutes of Health, 1987

What about taking drugs to lower my cholesterol?

Some people who have a high cholesterol level may not be able to lower it enough by diet changes alone. They may need to use a drug in addition to making changes in the way they eat. Drugs used most often are cholestyramine, colestipol and niacin.

Cholestyramine (Questran) and colestipol (Colestid) are resins that increase the excretion of cholesterol from the body. Major side effects are constipation, bloating and gas. They are unpleasant to take.

Niacin (nicotinic acid, a B vitamin) causes intense flushing and itching of the skin right after you take it. Major side effects are rashes and upset stomach. It can worsen diabetes and gout.

Lovastatin, a new drug approved by the FDA in late 1987, is recommended to be used with caution because there has not yet been time to evaluate its long-term effects. It is recommended for use when other drugs do not work.

COUNT UP
YOUR CHOLESTEROL

Most of us eat too much cholesterol each day.

We eat on the run and pick foods high in fat. By the end of the day we've eaten too much cholesterol.

You know that you shouldn't be eating a lot of cholesterol. You want to cut back. But it's not easy since you are not really sure which foods are high in cholesterol and which foods are not. With the *Cholesterol Counter* it's simple to find out which foods have cholesterol and to *count* the amount you are eating.

Let's look at a typical day. Are the food choices familiar? Let's see just how much cholesterol this sample day contains and how we can reduce the amount with better food choices.

CHOLESTEROL COUNTING:
A SAMPLE DAY OF POOR FOOD CHOICES

	CHOLESTEROL (MG)
Breakfast	
Orange juice (½ cup)	0
Scrambled eggs	427
Bacon (2 slices)	10
Toast (1 slice) &	0
Butter (1 tsp)	10
Coffee &	0
Cream (1 Tbsp)	6
Lunch	
Cheeseburger	
Hamburger (3 oz)	80
American cheese (1 slice)	25
Roll	0
Catsup	0
French fries	0
Vanilla shake	29
Snack	
Pound cake (1 slice)	46
Coffee &	0
Cream (1 Tbsp)	6
Dinner	
Batter-dipped fried chicken (½ breast)	119
Baked potato &	0
Sour cream (2 Tbsp)	14
Tossed salad &	0
Thousand Island dressing (¼ cup)	20
Apple pie (1 slice)	10
Tea &	0
Sugar	0
TV Snack	
Rich vanilla ice cream (1 cup)	88
TOTAL CHOLESTEROL:	890

This is too much cholesterol for one day—almost three times the recommended level of 300 milligrams a day. Now you can see how easy it is to take in more cholesterol than you need.

CHOLESTEROL COUNTING:
A SAMPLE DAY OF WISE FOOD CHOICES

	CHOLESTEROL (MG)
Breakfast	
Orange juice (4 oz)	0
All Bran &	
Lowfat milk (½ cup)	5
Toast (1 slice) &	0
Jelly	0
Coffee &	0
Lowfat milk (2 Tbsp)	1
Lunch	
Hamburger (3 oz)	80
Roll	0
Catsup	0
French fries	0
Cola	0
Snack	
Pear	0
Dinner	
Roasted chicken breast, no skin	
(½ breast)	73
Baked potato &	
Plain yogurt (2 Tbsp or 1 oz)	2
Tossed salad &	0
Oil & vinegar dressing (2 Tbsp)	0
Fruit cocktail (½ cup)	0
Tea &	0
Sugar	0
TV Snack	
Vanilla ice milk (1 cup)	18
TOTAL CHOLESTEROL:	179

Wise food choices! A much healthier intake of cholesterol for the day.

Now it's your turn to *count your cholesterol*. Note everything you eat today, then look up the cholesterol in each food you have eaten and see how much cholesterol you ate today. While you're at it, jot down the calories, too!

CHOLESTEROL COUNTING:
A SAMPLE WORKSHEET

FOOD	AMOUNT	CHOLESTEROL (MG)	CALORIES
Breakfast			
Snack			
Lunch			
Snack			
Dinner			
Snack			

TOTAL CHOLESTEROL: **CALORIES:**

Did your cholesterol total more than 300 milligrams for the day? If it did, you need to start counting cholesterol and making wiser food choices.

CHOLESTEROL COUNTING:
A SAMPLE WORKSHEET

FOOD	AMOUNT	CHOLESTEROL (MG)	CALORIES
Breakfast			
Snack			
Lunch			
Snack			
Dinner			
Snack			

TOTAL CHOLESTEROL: CALORIES:

Did your cholesterol total more than 300 milligrams for the day? If it did, you need to start counting cholesterol and making wiser food choices.

EIGHT STEPS
TO LOWER CHOLESTEROL

1. Use liquid vegetable oils. Choose olive, canola, corn, soybean, sunflower, safflower and cottonseed oils.

2. Limit amount of meat eaten. Do not use liver, brains or other organ meats. Poultry, shellfish and other fish also should be eaten in small portions.

3. Use lean cuts of meat; trim off all visible fat. Cook without added fat. Bake, broil or roast to further reduce fat. Remove skin from poultry and fish.

4. Use more beans, grains, pasta, rice and vegetables to make up for the smaller portions of meat, fish and poultry.

5. Avoid coffee whiteners (nondairy creamers) and whipped toppings.

6. Limit eggs to three a week, including those used in cooking and desserts. Two egg whites can be substituted for one egg.

7. Use skim milk, skim milk cheese, ice milk and lowfat yogurt. Avoid butter, cream, ice cream, sour cream and whole milk.

8. When using margarine, salad dressing or gravy, use a teaspoon or tablespoon to measure out a portion.

USING YOUR
CHOLESTEROL COUNTER

This book lists the cholesterol and calorie content of over 3000 foods. For the first time, information about cholesterol values is at your fingertips. Now you will find it easy to follow a low cholesterol diet.

Before *Cholesterol Counter* it was impossible to tell how much cholesterol there was in prepared foods since most do not list cholesterol information on the label. Fresh foods like meat, chicken, fish and cheese do not even have a label. The same goes for take-out items like potato salad, coleslaw, quiche, or foods bought at the bakery. How can you tell how much cholesterol there is in a burger or taco that you enjoy at the local fast food restaurant? *Cholesterol Counter* lists them all!

Foods are listed alphabetically, often grouped into categories like *candy, cereal* or *fish*. All categories are listed in the table of contents.

If you want to know how much cholesterol is in the tunafish sandwich you are having for lunch: (1) look under *FISH* or *SALAD*, where you will find tuna salad listed alphabetically in both places; (2) look under *BREAD & ROLLS*, where you will find the bread you are eating listed alphabetically. For foods like *FRENCH TOAST, HONEY* or *TAMALE*, that do not logically fit into a food category, simply look for the specific food alphabetically in the complete listing. For example, *FRENCH TOAST* is found on page 64, listed alphabetically between *FRENCH FRIES* and *FROG LEG*. Two slices have 224 milligrams of cholesterol.

Popular fast foods like *BURGER KING, DOMINO'S PIZZA,*

TACO BELL and *WENDY'S* are listed under the chain's name. For example *MCDONALD'S* is listed on page 92 under *M*.

If you are eating at home, simply look up the individual foods you are eating and total the cholesterol for the meal. For example, your dinner may consist of:

	CHOLESTEROL (MG)
2 rib lamb chops, broiled	132
Broccoli w/Cheese Sauce (Birds Eye)	5
Long Grain & Wild Rice (Minute Rice)	10
Pecan Pie (Mrs. Smith's)	30
Glass of white wine	0
TOTAL CHOLESTEROL FOR THE MEAL: 177	

We have tried to include all foods for which cholesterol values are known. There will be some foods, however, that are not listed in *Cholesterol Counter* because the cholesterol values are not available for that particular food.

When you can't locate your favorite brand, look at other foods in that category. You will probably find a similar brand food, a generic product or a home recipe that is like your favorite food. For example: You find that your favorite brand of vanilla yogurt is not listed. Ask yourself, "Is your favorite brand made from whole milk or is it lowfat?" If it is lowfat vanilla yogurt, on page 165 you will find a generic listing for lowfat vanilla yogurt as well as an entry for *Friendship Lowfat* vanilla yogurt and *Colombo Nonfat* vanilla yogurt. From these three entries you can quickly determine that lowfat vanilla yogurt has 14 milligrams or less cholesterol in a serving. You can then assume that your favorite brand has a comparable amount.

With your *Cholesterol Counter* as your guide, you will never again wonder how much cholesterol is in food. You will always be able to tell if a food is high in cholesterol, moderate in cholesterol or low in cholesterol. *Your goal is to pick low cholesterol foods each time you eat.*

Finding Cholesterol in the Foods You Eat

When you know the ingredients in a food you can tell if that food contains cholesterol. Read the ingredient list on the label or if you are making a homemade recipe read through the recipe ingredients. To find cholesterol-containing ingredients you need only remember this simple rule:

If it grows in the ground the food DOES NOT contain cholesterol.

If it has feet, fins, wings or claws and can walk, swim or fly, the food DOES contain cholesterol.

Try out the rule. Which of the following foods has cholesterol?

Is there cholesterol in:

	YES	NO
Hamburger	X	
Sardines	X	
Lobster	X	
Chicken leg	X	
Cheddar cheese	X	
Milk	X	
Egg	X	
Peanut butter		X
Apple		X
Olive oil		X

The first seven foods all contain cholesterol. Hamburger comes from a steer. Sardines and lobsters are seafood. Chicken leg comes from a chicken. All of these have either feet, fins, wings or claws. Therefore, they all contain cholesterol. Cheddar cheese, milk and egg have cholesterol because they all come from an animal that has feet.

Peanut butter, apples and olive oil are all from plants that grow in the ground. Therefore, they have no cholesterol.

Now you know why all of the ingredients on the following list have cholesterol. These are the ingredients to look for on a label or in a recipe.

INGREDIENTS THAT CONTAIN CHOLESTEROL
whole eggs
egg yolks
whole milk
lowfat milk
cream
ice cream
sour cream
yogurt (unless labeled nonfat)
cheese (unless labeled nonfat)
bacon or bacon fat
butter
lard
chicken fat
beef suet or tallow
liver
kidney
brains
meat (any variety)
fish (any variety)
poultry (any variety)

Here are some sample labels with the cholesterol containing ingredients highlighted.

KEEBLER STONE CREEK HEARTY RYE CRACKERS
Enriched wheat flour containing niacin, reduced iron, thiamine mononitrate (vitamin B1) and riboflavin (vitamin B2), *animal* or vegetable shortening (*lard* or partially hydrogenated soybean oil), sugar, stone ground rye flour, stone ground corn flour, salt, molasses, dehydrated onion, leavening, spices, artificial color (caramel) and lecithin.

These crackers have only one ingredient that contains cholesterol, but it is the second ingredient listed after flour. This means that the crackers contain more lard or soybean oil than any other ingredient except flour. Note that lard *or* soybean oil may be used. You have no way of knowing which was used. It is safer to assume it is the lard and that the crackers contain cholesterol.

NOODLE RONI CHICKEN AND MUSHROOM FLAVOR
Egg noodles, food starch modified, natural flavors, *chicken fat,* hydrolyzed vegetable protein with dry yeast and soy flour, dried mushrooms, *dried chicken,* monosodium glutamate, dried onion, dried red pepper, onion, turmeric, tricalcium phosphate, sugar, dried parsley, spice, dried garlic, disodium inosinate, disodium guanylate, freshness preserved with BHA, propylgallate, citric acid.

This side dish contains three sources of cholesterol: egg, chicken fat and dried chicken.

FRENCH'S IDAHO MASHED POTATOES
Idaho potato granules (with sodium bisulfite, citric acid and BHA added to protect color and flavor), monoglycerides.

Although these instant mashed potatoes contain no cholesterol, the package directions tell you to add butter and milk. *Both are sources of cholesterol.* Even though you buy a cholesterol-free product, you may be adding cholesterol in the preparation.

To cut down on the cholesterol in the instant mashed potatoes, you could use skim milk and margarine in place of butter and whole milk.

DEFINITIONS

as prepared: refers to food that has been prepared according to package directions

cooked: refers to food cooked without the addition of fat (oil, butter, margarine, etc.); steaming, poaching, broiling and dry roasting are examples of this type of preparation

fully trimmed: describes meat that has had all the fat cut off its edges or poultry that has had all fat and skin cut off

generic: describes a food without a brand name

home recipe: describes homemade dishes; those included can be used as guide to the cholesterol and calorie values of similar products you may prepare or take-out food you buy ready-to-eat

not trimmed: describes meat with some fat on its edges that is not cut away before cooking or poultry prepared with skin and fat as purchased

ABBREVIATIONS

avg	=	average
diam	=	diameter
frzn	=	frozen
g	=	gram
lb	=	pound
lg	=	large
med	=	medium
mg	=	milligram
oz	=	ounce
pkg	=	package
prep	=	prepared
reg	=	regular
sm	=	small
sq	=	square
Tbsp	=	tablespoon
tr	=	trace
tsp	=	teaspoon
w/	=	with
w/o	=	without
"	=	inch
<	=	less than

EQUIVALENT MEASURES

1 tablespoon	=	3 teaspoons
4 tablespoons	=	¼ cup
8 tablespoons	=	½ cup
12 tablespoons	=	¾ cup
16 tablespoons	=	1 cup

| 1000 milligrams | = | 1 gram |
| 28 grams | = | 1 ounce |

LIQUID MEASUREMENTS			DRY MEASUREMENTS		
2 tablespoons	=	1 ounce	16 ounces	=	1 pound
¼ cup	=	2 ounces	12 ounces	=	¾ pound
½ cup	=	4 ounces	8 ounces	=	½ pound
¾ cup	=	6 ounces	4 ounces	=	¼ pound
1 cup	=	8 ounces			
2 cups	=	1 pint			
4 cups	=	1 quart			

THE
CHOLESTEROL
COUNTER

FOOD	PORTION SIZE	CALORIES	CHOLESTEROL (Mg)
ARBY'S			
Bac'n Cheddar Deluxe	1	561	78
Baked Potato, Plain	1	290	none
Beef'n Cheddar	1	490	51
Chicken Breast Sandwich	1	592	57
Chicken Club Sandwich	1	621	108
Chicken Salad & Croissant	1	472	12
Chicken Salad Sandwich	1	386	30
Chicken Salad w/Tomato & Lettuce	1	515	12
Chocolate Shake	1	384	32
French Fries	1 portion	211	6
Hot Ham 'n Cheese	1	353	50
Jamocha Shake	1	424	31
King Roast Beef	1	467	49
Potato Cakes	2	201	1
Roast Beef, deluxe	1	486	59
Roast Beef, jr	1	218	20
Roast Beef, reg	1	350	39
Roast Beef, super	1	501	40
Roasted Chicken Breast	1	254	200
Roasted Chicken Leg	1	319	214
Superstuffed Potato, Broccoli and Cheddar	1	541	24
Superstuffed Potato, Deluxe	1	648	72
Superstuffed Potato, Mushroom and Cheese	1	506	21
Superstuffed Potato, Taco	1	619	145
Tossed Salad, Plain	1 portion	44	none
Tossed Salad, w/20 Calorie Italian Dressing	1 portion	57	none
Turkey Deluxe	1	375	39
Vanilla Shake	1	295	30

FOOD	PORTION SIZE	CALORIES	CHOLESTEROL (Mg)

BACON

FOOD	PORTION SIZE	CALORIES	CHOLESTEROL (Mg)
Bacon; cooked (Generic)	2 strips (½ oz)	70	10
Bacon; cooked (Oscar Mayer)	1 strip (6 g)	35	5
Bacon, Center Cut; cooked (Oscar Mayer)	1 strip (4.6 g)	24	5
Bacon, Sliced; cooked (Farmland Foods, Inc)	3½ strips (1 oz)	160	17
Bacon, Thick Sliced; cooked (Oscar Mayer)	1 strip (11 g)	64	10
Bacon, *West Virginia;* cooked (Hygrade's)	3–4 strips	154	19
Bacon Bits (Oscar Mayer)	1½ tsp	21	6
Bacon Fat	1 Tbsp	135	14
Bacos (General Mills)	1 Tbsp	36	none
Breakfast Strips, Beef, *Lean 'N Tasty* (Oscar Mayer)	1 heated strip	46	13
Breakfast Strips, Pork, *Lean 'N Tasty* (Oscar Mayer)	1 heated strip	52	14
Canadian bacon; broiled or fried (Generic)	2 strips (42 g)	116	37
Canadian Style Bacon; cooked (Oscar Mayer)	1 strip (28 g)	35	12
Sizzlean, Pork; cooked (Swift)	2 strips	70	20
Sizzlean, Premium; cooked (Swift)	3–4 strips (1 oz)	123	35
Sizzlean/Firebrand; cooked (Swift)	2 strips	50	15

BAKING POWDER

FOOD	PORTION SIZE	CALORIES	CHOLESTEROL (Mg)
Calumet (General Foods)	1 Tbsp	2	none

FOOD	PORTION SIZE	CALORIES	CHOLESTEROL (Mg)
BAKING SODA			
Arm & Hammer (Church & Dwight Co.)	1 tsp	0	none
BEANS (*see also* VEGETABLES)			
Baked, canned, w/beef (Generic)	½ cup	161	29
Baked, canned, w/franks (Generic)	½ cup	182	8
Baked, canned, w/pork (Generic)	½ cup	133	9
Baked, canned, w/pork & tomato sauce (Generic)	½ cup	123	9
Baked, canned, w/pork & sweet sauce (Generic)	½ cup	140	9
Baked beans (Home recipe)	½ cup	190	6
Chickpeas, canned (Generic)	½ cup	143	none
Cowpeas, w/pork, canned (Generic)	½ cup	99	8
Falafel (Home recipe)	1 patty (½ oz)	57	none
Hummus (Home recipe)	⅓ cup	140	none
Kidney, canned (Generic)	½ cup	104	none
Lentils; boiled (Generic)	½ cup	115	none
Lima beans, canned (Generic)	½ cup	95	none
Navy, canned (Generic)	½ cup	148	none
Pinto, canned (Generic)	½ cup	93	none
Split peas; cooked (Generic)	½ cup	116	none

FOOD	PORTION SIZE	CALORIES	CHOLESTEROL (Mg)

BEEF
(*see also* VEAL)

FOOD	PORTION SIZE	CALORIES	CHOLESTEROL (Mg)
Brisket, w/o bone, fully trimmed; cooked	3 slices 5 × 1 × ¼" each	167	68
Brisket, w/o bone, not trimmed; cooked	3 slices 5 × 1 × ¼" each	356	71
Chuck roast, w/o bone, fully trimmed; braised	1 slice 3 × 2 × ¾"	164	77
Chuck roast, w/o bone, not trimmed; braised	1 slice 3 × 2 × ¾"	246	80
Chuck steak, w/bone, fully trimmed; braised	7 oz	266	97
Chuck steak, w/bone, not trimmed; braised	7 oz	534	118
Chuck stew meat, w/o bone, fully trimmed; braised	5 cubes 1" each	182	77
Chuck stew meat, w/o bone, fully trimmed, cubed; braised	½ cup	162	69
Chuck stew meat, w/o bone, not trimmed, cubed; braised	½ cup	247	71
Club steak, w/bone, fully trimmed	10 oz raw	198	74
Club steak, w/bone, not trimmed	8 oz raw	631	131
Corned beef; cooked	1 slice 5 × 1 × ¼"	104	26
Corned beef; canned (Generic)	1 slice 3 × 2 × ¼"	60	26
Corned beef & egg casserole (Home recipe)	¾ cup	278	159

FOOD	PORTION SIZE	CALORIES	CHOLESTEROL (Mg)
Cube steak, fully trimmed; cooked	4 × 2½ × ½"	222	80
Dry beef; creamed (Home recipe)	⅔ cup	211	32
Flank steak, w/o bone, not trimmed; braised	2½" sq × ¾" (3 oz)	167	77
Ground round, fully trimmed; cooked	½ cup	104	50
Ground round, fully trimmed; cooked	3" diam × ⅝" patty	161	77
Ground round, not trimmed; cooked	½ cup	144	52
Ground round, not trimmed; cooked	3" diam × ⅝" patty	227	82
Ground sirloin, fully trimmed; cooked	½ cup	114	50
Ground sirloin, not trimmed; cooked	½ cup	213	52
Hamburger casserole (Home recipe)	¾ cup	205	63
Hamburger Helper, Beef Noodle; as prep	1 serving	326	61
Hamburger Helper, Cheeseburger Macaroni; as prep	1 serving	366	61
Hamburger Helper, Chili Tomato; as prep	1 serving	336	61
Hamburger Helper, Lasagne; as prep	1 serving	336	61
Hamburger patty; cooked	3" diam × ⅝"	243	80
Italian loaf (Home recipe)	1 slice 3" sq × ¾"	234	94
Minute steak; cooked	4 × 2½ × ½"	222	80

FOOD	PORTION SIZE	CALORIES	CHOLESTEROL (Mg)
Porterhouse steak, w/bone, not trimmed	1 lb raw	1400	283
Porterhouse steak, w/bone, fully trimmed	1 lb raw	385	157
Porterhouse steak, w/o bone, fully trimmed; broiled	4 × 3 × ½″ (3 oz)	190	77
Porterhouse steak, w/o bone, not trimmed; broiled	4 × 3 × ½″ (3 oz)	395	80
Potpie; baked (Home recipe)	4¼″ pie	558	48
Rib roast, fully trimmed; cooked, chopped	½ cup	169	64
Rib roast, w/o bone, fully trimmed; roasted	2 slices 5 × 2 × ¼″ each	200	76
Rib roast, w/o bone, not trimmed; cooked	2 slices 5 × 2 × ¼″ each	365	78
Rib steak, w/bone, fully trimmed	½ lb raw	292	110
Rib steak, w/bone, not trimmed	1 lb raw	1008	215
Rib steak, w/o bone, fully trimmed; broiled	4 × 3 × ½″ (3 oz)	205	77
Rib steak, w/o bone, not trimmed; broiled	4″ sq × ½″ (3 oz)	374	80
Roast beef, canned (Generic)	3 slices 3 × 2 × ¼″ each	188	76
Round steak, w/o bone, fully trimmed; braised	4 × 3 × ½″ (3 oz)	161	77
Round steak, w/o bone, not trimmed; braised	4 × 3 × ½″ (3 oz)	222	80
Rump roast, w/o bone, fully trimmed; cooked, chopped	½ cup	146	64

FOOD	PORTION SIZE	CALORIES	CHOLESTEROL (Mg)
Rump roast, w/o bone, fully trimmed; cooked	2 slices 5 × 2 × ¼" each	173	76
Rump roast, w/o bone, not trimmed; cooked	2 slices 5 × 2 × ⅛" each	288	78
Sauerbraten; cooked (Home recipe)	1 slice 3 × 2 × ¾"	190	75
Short ribs, not trimmed; cooked	2 med ribs	645	128
Sirloin steak, w/bone, fully trimmed	½ lb raw	211	93
Sirloin steak, w/bone, not trimmed	½ lb raw	596	145
Sirloin steak, w/o bone, fully trimmed; broiled	4 × 3 × ½" (3 oz)	176	77
Sirloin steak, w/o bone, not trimmed; broiled	4 × 3 × ½" (3 oz)	329	80
Sirloin tip, fully trimmed; roasted, chopped	½ cup	168	64
Sirloin tip, fully trimmed; roasted	2 slices (3 oz)	204	77
Sirloin tip, not trimmed; roasted	2 slices (3 oz)	414	80
Steakette, w/o bone	2 oz raw	103	37
Strip steak, w/o bone, fully trimmed	8 oz raw	335	137
Strip steak, w/o bone, not trimmed; broiled	4 × 3 × ½"	412	82
Stroganoff (Home recipe)	¾ cup	260	69
Swiss steak (Home recipe)	3 × 3 × ½" piece	214	61

FOOD	PORTION SIZE	CALORIES	CHOLESTEROL (Mg)
T-bone steak, w/bone, fully trimmed	10 oz raw	248	101
T-bone steak, w/bone, not trimmed	10 oz raw	941	187
T-bone steak, w/o bone, fully trimmed; broiled	4 × 3 × ½" (3 oz)	190	77
T-bone steak, w/o bone, not trimmed; broiled	4 × 3 × ½" (3 oz)	402	80
Tenderloin steak, w/o bone, fully trimmed; broiled	3¼"sq × ¾" (4 oz)	263	107

BEER
(*see also* LIQUOR/LIQUEURS, WINE)

FOOD	PORTION SIZE	CALORIES	CHOLESTEROL (Mg)
Ale	12 oz	155	none
Anheuser Busch Natural Light	12 oz	110	none
Beer, 4.5% alcohol	12 oz	155	none
Bud Light	12 oz	108	none
Coors Light	12 oz	105	none
Guiness Kaliber, nonalcoholic beer	12 oz	43	none
Michelob Light	12 oz	134	none
Miller Lite	12 oz	96	none
Molson Light	12 oz	109	none
Schlitz Light	12 oz	96	none
Schmidts Light	12 oz	96	none
Stroh Light	12 oz	115	none

BEVERAGES, ALCOHOLIC
(*see* BEER, LIQUOR/LIQUEURS, WINE)

FOOD	PORTION SIZE	CALORIES	CHOLESTEROL (Mg)

BEVERAGES, NONALCOHOLIC
(*see* COFFEE/TEA, FRUIT DRINKS, MILK, MILK DRINKS, MINERAL WATER, SODA)

BOLOGNA
(*see* LUNCHEON MEAT/COLD CUTS, TURKEY)

BRAINS

FOOD	PORTION SIZE	CALORIES	CHOLESTEROL (Mg)
Beef; cooked (Generic)	3 oz	136	1746
Pork; cooked (Generic)	3 oz	117	2169

BREAD & ROLLS
(*see also* TORTILLA)

FOOD	PORTION SIZE	CALORIES	CHOLESTEROL (Mg)
Bagels, egg (Generic)	1 bagel	126	26
Bagles, plain (Lender's)	1 bagel (2 oz)	150	none
Biscuit (Generic)	1	90	none
Bread, banana (Home recipe)	1 slice 3 × 2½ × ½″	116	25
Bread, bran raisin (Generic)	1 lg slice	151	none
Bread, cracked wheat (Generic)	1 slice	66	none
Bread Crumbs, Seasoned (Contadina)	1 Tbsp	35	<1
Bread, French (Generic)	1 slice 4¾ × 4 × ½″	73	none
Bread, *Honey Wheat Berry* (Arnold)	2 slices	180	<5

FOOD	PORTION SIZE	CALORIES	CHOLESTEROL (Mg)
Bread, Italian (Generic)	1 slice 5 × 3 × ¾"	88	none
Bread, nut (Home recipe)	1 slice	127	13
Bread, Pumpernickle (Arnold)	2 slices	150	none
Bread, Pumpernickle, dark rye (Generic)	1 slice	62	none
Bread, Pumpernickle, dark rye, snack loaf (Generic)	1 sm slice	17	none
Bread, pumpkin (Home recipe)	1 slice	127	38
Bread, raisin (Generic)	1 slice (25g)	66	none
Bread, raisin (Home recipe)	1 slice (45g)	140	6
Bread, *Roman Meal* (Ralston Purina)	2 slices	140	<5
Bread, rye, light (Generic)	1 slice	61	none
Bread, rye, light, snack loaf (Generic)	1 sm slice	17	none
Bread, Vienna (Generic)	1 slice	73	none
Bread, Wheat, *Fresh Horizons* (Ralston Purina)	2 slices	100	none
Bread, White, *Brick Oven* (Arnold)	2 slices	130	<5
Bread, white, enriched; toasted (Generic)	1 slice	68	none
Bread, White, *Fresh Horizons* (Ralston Purina)	2 slices	100	none
Bread, White, *Home Pride Butter Top* (Ralston Purina)	2 slices	150	<5
Bread, White, Thin Slice (Weight Watchers)	1 thin slice	35	none
Bread, whole wheat (Generic)	1 slice	56	1
Bread, Whole Wheat, *Brick Oven* (Arnold)	2 slices	120	<5

FOOD	PORTION SIZE	CALORIES	CHOLESTEROL (Mg)
Bread, Whole Wheat 100%, *Home Pride* (Ralston Purina)	2 slices	140	<5
Croissant, *Colonial Wheat* (Rainbo)	1	300	5
Crouton, *Croutettes* (Kellogg's)	½ cup	72	none
English Muffin (Thomas)	1	130	none
English Muffin, *Honey Wheat* (Thomas)	1	129	none
Muffin, apple (Home recipe)	1	137	21
Muffin, blueberry (Home recipe)	1	147	22
Muffin, Blueberry Muffin Mix, *Bakery Style;* as prep (Duncan Hines)	1	190	10
Muffin, Blueberry Muffin, Wild; as prep (Duncan Hines)	1	110	20
Muffin, Blueberry Muffin, Wild; as prep (Betty Crocker)	1	120	20
Muffin, bran (Home recipe)	1	104	21
Muffin, Bran & Honey Muffin Mix; as prep (Duncan Hines)	1	120	7
Muffin, Bran & Honey Nut Muffin Mix, *Bakery Style;* as prep (Duncan Hines)	1	200	10
Muffin, Bran Date Muffin, *Jiffy;* as prep (Chelsea Milling Co.)	1	110	10
Muffin, Cinnamon Swirl Muffin Mix, *Bakery Style;* as prep (Duncan Hines)	1	200	10
Muffin, corn (Home recipe)	1	169	40
Muffin, Corn Muffin Mix; as prep (Betty Crocker)	1	160	20
Muffin, Corn Muffin Mix, *Jiffy;* as prep (Chelsea Milling Co.)	1	115	10

FOOD	PORTION SIZE	CALORIES	CHOLESTEROL (Mg)
Muffin, *Hearty Fruit Muffin*, frzn, any flavor (Sara Lee)	1 (2¼ oz)	220	none
Muffin, orange (Home recipe)	1	137	33
Muffin, Pecan Nut Muffin Mix, *Bakery Style;* as prep (Duncan Hines)	1	220	10
Muffin, plain (Home recipe)	1	158	25
Muffin, whole wheat (Home recipe)	1	123	31
Pita (Generic)	1 pocket	182	none
Popover (Home recipe)	1	98	61
Roll, hamburger (Generic)	1	114	none
Roll, hard (Generic)	1	93	1
Roll, Hot Dog (Arnold)	1	110	none
Roll, Hot Roll Mix; as prep (Pillsbury)	2	240	18
Scones (Home recipe)	1	130	56
Sourdough (Home recipe)	1 slice	76	none
Yorkshire pudding (Home recipe)	3" sq	171	86

BREAKFAST BARS
(*see* NUTRITIONAL SUPPLEMENTS)

BURGER KING

Apple Pie	1	305	4
Bacon Double Cheeseburger	1	510	104
B'kfast Croissanwich, Bacon, Egg, Cheese	1	355	249
B'kfast Croissanwich, Ham, Egg, Cheese	1	335	262

FOOD	PORTION SIZE	CALORIES	CHOLESTEROL (Mg)
B'kfast Croissanwich, Sausage, Egg, Cheese	1	538	293
Cheeseburger	1	317	48
Cherry Pie	1	357	6
Chicken Sandwich	1	688	82
Chicken Tenders	1	204	47
French Fries, reg	1	227	14
French Toast Platter w/Bacon	1	469	73
French Toast Platter w/Sausage	1	635	115
Ham & Cheese	1	471	70
Hamburger	1	275	37
Onion Rings, reg	1	274	none
Pecan Pie	1	459	4
Salad Plain	1	28	none
Salad, w/Bleu Cheese	1	184	22
Salad, w/French	1	152	none
Salad, w/Golden Italian	1	162	none
Salad, w/House Dressing	1	159	11
Salad, w/Reduced Calorie Italian	1	42	none
Salad, w/1000 Island	1	145	17
Scrambled Egg Platter	1	468	370
Scrambled Egg Platter w/Bacon	1	536	378
Scrambled Egg Platter w/ Sausage	1	702	420
Whaler Fish Sandwich	1	488	84
Whaler w/Cheese	1	530	95
Whopper Junior	1	370	41
Whopper Junior w/Cheese	1	420	52
Whopper Sandwich	1	640	94
Whopper w/Cheese	1	723	117

FOOD	PORTION SIZE	CALORIES	CHOLESTEROL (Mg)

BUTTER
(*see also* FATS, MARGARINE, MAYONNAISE, NUTS, OILS, PEANUT BUTTER)

FOOD	PORTION SIZE	CALORIES	CHOLESTEROL (Mg)
Butter Buds (Cumberland)	2 Tbsp (1 oz)	12	none
Molly McButter All Natural Butter Flavor Sprinkles (Alberto-Culver)	½ tsp	4	none
Regular (Generic)	1 Tbsp	102	31
Regular, Lightly Salted Sweet Cream (Land O Lakes)	1 Tbsp	100	30
Regular, unsalted (Generic)	1 Tbsp	102	31
Regular, Unsalted Sweet Cream (Land O Lakes)	1 Tbsp	100	30
Whipped, Lightly Salted Sweet Cream (Land O Lakes)	1 Tbsp	60	20
Whipped, Unsalted (Land O Lakes)	1 Tbsp	60	20

BUTTER BLENDS
(*see* MARGARINE)

CAKE
(*see also* COOKIES, DOUGHNUTS, PIE, QUICHE)

FOOD	PORTION SIZE	CALORIES	CHOLESTEROL (Mg)
Angel food (Home recipe)	1 piece (2 oz)	161	none
Apple (Home recipe)	2" sq	145	21
Baklava (Home recipe)	1½" sq	126	23
Boston cream (Home recipe)	⅛ of 9" cake	433	158
Carrot, w/cream cheese icing (Home recipe)	2 × 2 × 1¾"	80	45

FOOD	PORTION SIZE	CALORIES	CHOLESTEROL (Mg)
Cheese cake (Home recipe)	⅛ of 8″ cake	414	159
Cheesecake; as prep w/whole milk (Jello-O)	⅛ of 8″ cake	280	30
Cheese, Cherry French Cream, frzn (Sara Lee)	1 piece (3 oz)	254	68
Chocolate or devil's food mix (Generic)	⅙ of 9″ cake	287	57
Chocolate or devil's food, w/ chocolate icing (Generic)	3 × 4″	350	64
Coffee cake, iced (Home recipe)	3″ sq	341	35
Coffee cake, nuts & icing (Generic)	3″ sq	372	35
Danish pastry, plain (Home recipe)	4¼″ diam	294	96
Donut, Cinnamon Apple (Earth Grains)	1	310	25
Donut, Devil's Food (Earth Grains)	1	330	20
Donut, Old Fashioned, Glazed (Earth Grains)	1	310	20
Donut, Old Fashioned, Powdered (Earth Grains)	1	290	20
Fruit cake, dark (Home recipe)	1½″ sq	163	19
Gingerbread (Home recipe)	3″ sq	276	28
Hostess Devil's Food Cupcake	1 cake	136	4
Hostess Hoho	1 cake	119	13
Hostess Snoball	1 cake	136	2
Hostess Twinkie	1 cake	144	21
Lady finger	1	40	39
Little Debbie Snak Cake, Apple Delight	1.17 oz	130	none
Little Debbie Snak Cake, Butterscotch Cakes	2.4 oz	310	none

FOOD	PORTION SIZE	CALORIES	CHOLESTEROL (Mg)
Little Debbie Snak Cake, Chocolate Cakes	2.4 oz	310	none
Little Debbie Snak Cake, Chocolate Snack Pastry	3.0 oz	390	none
Little Debbie Snak Cake, Dutch Apple	2.5 oz	270	none
Little Debbie Snak Cake, Fudge Brownie	3.0 oz	350	none
Little Debbie Snak Cake, Fudge Crispy	1.3 oz	170	none
Little Debbie Snak Cake, Lemon Stik	1.5 oz	220	none
Little Debbie Snak Cake, Marshmallow Pies	1.2 oz	150	none
Little Debbie Snak Cake, Oatmeal Creme Pie	1.8 oz	350	none
Little Debbie Snak Cake, Peanut Butter Bar	2.0 oz	290	none
Little Debbie Snak Cake, Pecan Pie	1.8 oz	170	none
Little Debbie Snak Cake, Swiss Roll	2.3 oz	280	none
Oatmeal cake, iced (Home recipe)	3" sq	356	74
Peanut butter cake (Home recipe)	3" sq	211	22
Pound cake (Home recipe)	3" sq	119	46
Scones (Home recipe)	1	130	56
Spice cake, w/caramel icing (Generic)	3" sq	411	61
Sponge cake (Home recipe)	3" sq	135	48
Strudel (Home recipe)	2½" sq	273	39
Torte, chocolate (Home recipe)	1" wedge	317	61
White cake (Home recipe)	3" sq	273	3

FOOD	PORTION SIZE	CALORIES	CHOLESTEROL (Mg)
White cake, w/uncooked white icing (Generic)	3″ sq	481	19
Yellow cake (Home recipe)	3″ sq	321	43
Yellow cake, w/chocolate icing (Home recipe)	3″ sq	463	69

CAKE MIX

FOOD	PORTION SIZE	CALORIES	CHOLESTEROL (Mg)
Aunt Jemima, Easy Mix Coffee Cake; as prep	⅛ cake	170	12
Duncan Hines, Angel Food; as prep	¹⁄₁₂ cake	140	none
Duncan Hines, Banana Bread; as prep	¹⁄₁₂ bread	160	7
Duncan Hines, Butter Recipe, Golden; as prep	¹⁄₁₂ cake	270	90
Duncan Hines, Chocolate; as prep	¹⁄₁₂ cake	280	70
Duncan Hines, Devil's Food Lite; as prep	¹⁄₁₂ cake	203	46
Duncan Hines, Devil's Food Original; as prep	¹⁄₁₂ cake	280	69
Duncan Hines, Lemon Supreme; as prep	¹⁄₁₂ cake	260	70
Duncan Hines, Marble Fudge; as prep	¹⁄₁₂ cake	260	70
Duncan Hines, Nut Bread; as prep	¹⁄₁₂ bread	170	7
Duncan Hines, Strawberry Supreme; as prep	¹⁄₁₂ cake	260	70
Duncan Hines, White; as prep	¹⁄₁₂ cake	250	70
Duncan Hines, Yellow Original; as prep	¹⁄₁₂ cake	260	69

FOOD	PORTION SIZE	CALORIES	CHOLESTEROL (Mg)
Pillsbury, Microwave Yellow Cake Mix; as prep	⅛ cake	220	10

CANDY
(*see also* CHOCOLATE/COCOA)

FOOD	PORTION SIZE	CALORIES	CHOLESTEROL (Mg)
Almonds, chocolate covered (Generic)	¼ cup	235	4
Bar, chocolate coated coconut center (Generic)	1 oz bar	124	tr
Bar, chocolate coated honeycomb w/peanut butter (Generic)	1 oz bar	131	tr
Bar, chocolate, plain (Generic)	1 oz bar	148	4
Bar, chocolate w/almonds (Generic)	1 oz bar	151	4
Bar, chocolate w/peanuts (Generic)	1 oz bar	154	3
Bar, *Crunch* (Nestle)	1¹⁄₁₆ oz	160	5
Bar, *KIT KAT Wafer* (Hershey)	3½ oz (100g)	530	25
Bar, *Krackel*, Chocolate (Hershey)	3½ oz	530	20
Bar, Milk Chocolate (Hershey)	3½ oz	540	25
Bar, Milk Chocolate, Almonds (Hershey's)	3½ oz	560	27
Bar, peanut (Generic)	1 oz bar	146	none
Bar, *Special Dark* (Hershey)	3½ oz (100g)	540	8
Bridge Mix (Nabisco)	1 oz	126	tr
Candy corn (Generic)	¼ cup	182	none
Caramel (Generic)	1 sq	40	none

FOOD	PORTION SIZE	CALORIES	CHOLESTEROL (Mg)
Caramels in Milk Chocolate, *Rolo* (Hershey)	1.93 oz pkg (10 pieces)	262	13
Caramels in Milk Chocolate, *Rolo* (Hershey)	3½ oz	480	23
Chocolate chips, chocolate flavored (Generic)	¼ cup	195	tr
Chocolate chips, milk chocolate (Generic)	¼ cup	218	7
Chocolate Chunks (Saco)	17g (6 pieces)	80	none
Fruit, candied, cherry (Generic)	1 cherry	12	none
Hershey's Kisses (Hershey)	20 Kisses (100g)	540	25
Jelly beans (Generic)	¼ cup	202	0
Licorice (Generic)	1 stick	35	none
Lollipop or sucker (Generic)	1 oz sucker	110	tr
Malted milk ball, chocolate coated (Generic)	1 ball	25	1
Malted Milk Tablets, Chocolate (Horlicks)	1 tablet	5	none
Malted Milk Tablets, Natural (Horlicks)	1 tablet	5	none
Marshmallow (Generic)	1	25	none
Milk Chocolate Bar w/Almonds (Hershey)	3½ oz	560	27
Mr. Goodbar (Hershey)	1.27 oz	198	5
Mr. Goodbar (Hershey)	1.65 oz	250	7
Mr. Goodbar (Hershey)	2 oz	300	8
Peanut brittle (Generic)	1 oz	120	none
Peanut Butter Chips, *Reese's* (Hershey)	3½ oz	530	6.1
Peanut Butter Cup, *Reese's* (Hershey)	2 pieces	184	5

FOOD	PORTION SIZE	CALORIES	CHOLESTEROL (Mg)
Peanut Butter Cups, *Reese's* (Hershey)	1 snack size	91	2.5
Peanut Butter Cups, *Reese's* (Hershey)	6 snack size	550	15.1
Peanuts, chocolate covered (Generic)	1 oz	159	3
Peppermint pattie, chocolate covered (Generic)	1 oz bar	116	tr
Peppermint Pattie, Chocolate Covered (Nabisco)	1	64	tr
Raisins, chocolate covered (Generic)	1 oz	121	2
Reese's Pieces (Hershey)	3½ oz	490	4
Thin Mint (Nabisco)	1	42	tr
Tootsie Roll, Miniature	1 sm	24	none

CARNATION SLENDER
(*see* NUTRITIONAL SUPPLEMENTS)

CATSUP

FOOD	PORTION SIZE	CALORIES	CHOLESTEROL (Mg)
Del Monte Tomato catsup	1 Tbsp	15	none
Heinz Ketchup	1 Tbsp	18	none
Heinz Low Sodium, *Lite* Ketchup	1 Tbsp	8	none
Tillie Lewis Catsup, Low Sodium, Low Calorie	1 Tbsp	8	none

CAVIAR
(*see* FISH)

FOOD	PORTION SIZE	CALORIES	CHOLESTEROL (Mg)

CEREAL

Cereals do not contain cholesterol unless they are served with milk, butter or cream.

FOOD	PORTION SIZE	CALORIES	CHOLESTEROL (Mg)
All Bran; w/½ cup whole milk (Kellogg's)	⅓ cup	140	16
All-Bran; w/½ cup lowfat milk (Kellogg's)	⅓ cup	115	5
All-Bran; w/½ cup skim milk (Kellogg's)	⅓ cup	108	2
Alpha-Bits; w/½ cup whole milk (General Foods)	1 cup	190	16
Alpha-Bits; w/½ cup lowfat milk (General Foods)	1 cup	165	5
Alpha-Bits; w/½ cup skim milk (General Foods)	1 cup	158	2
Apple Jacks; w/½ cup whole milk (Kellogg's)	1 cup	180	16
Apple Jacks; w/½ cup lowfat milk (Kellogg's)	1 cup	149	5
Apple Jacks; w/½ cup skim milk (Kellogg's)	1 cup	142	2
Cap'n Crunch's Crunchberries w/½ cup whole milk (Quaker)	1 cup	200	16
Cap'n Crunch's Crunchberries w/½ cup lowfat milk (Quaker)	1 cup	175	5
Cap'n Crunch's Crunchberries; w/½ cup skim milk (Quaker)	1 cup	168	2
Cap'n Crunch; w/½ cup whole milk (Quaker)	1 cup	201	16
Cap'n Crunch; w/½ cup lowfat milk (Quaker)	1 cup	176	5

FOOD	PORTION SIZE	CALORIES	CHOLESTEROL (Mg)
Cap'n Crunch; w/½ cup skim milk (Quaker)	1 cup	169	2
Cheerios; w/½ cup whole milk (General Mills)	1¼ cup	190	16
Cherrios; w/½ cup lowfat milk (General Mills)	1¼ cup	165	5
Cheerios; w/½ cup skim milk (General Mills)	1¼ cup	158	2
Cocoa Krispies; w/½ cup whole milk (Kellogg's)	¾ cup	190	16
Cocoa Krispies; w/½ cup lowfat milk (Kellogg's)	¾ cup	165	5
Cocoa Krispies; w/½ cup skim milk (Kellogg's)	¾ cup	158	2
Natural Valley Granola; w/½ cup whole milk (General Foods)	⅓ cup	201	16
Natural Valley Granola; w/½ cup lowfat milk (General Foods)	⅓ cup	181	5
Nature Valley Granola; w/½ cup skim milk (General Foods)	⅓ cup	166	2
Nutri-Grain; corn; w/½ cup whole milk (Kellogg's)	⅔ cup	188	16
Nutri-Grain; corn; w/½ cup lowfat milk (Kellogg's)	⅔ cup	163	5
Nutri-Grain; corn; w/½ cup skim milk (Kellogg's)	⅔ cup	148	2
Oatmeal; cooked, w/¼ cup whole milk (Generic)	¾ cup	165	8
Oatmeal; cooked, w/¼ cup lowfat milk (Generic)	¾ cup	153	3
Oatmeal; cooked, w/¼ cup skim milk (Generic)	¾ cup	148	1

FOOD	PORTION SIZE	CALORIES	CHOLESTEROL (Mg)

CHEESE, NATURAL
(*see also* CHEESE, PROCESSED; CHEESE DISHES; CREAM CHEESE)

FOOD	PORTION SIZE	CALORIES	CHOLESTEROL (Mg)
Blue (Frigo)	1 oz	100	21
Blue (Generic)	1 oz	100	21
Blue (Generic)	1 Tbsp	30	6
Blue (Kraft)	1 oz	100	30
Blue, *Roka Brand* (Kraft)	1 oz	70	20
Brick (Generic)	1 oz	105	27
Brick (Kraft)	1 oz	110	30
Brick (Land O Lakes)	1 oz	110	25
Brie (Generic)	⅔ × 1 × 1″	95	28
Camembert (Generic)	⅓ oz pkg	114	27
Caraway (Kraft)	1 oz	100	30
Cheddar (Generic)	1 cup	455	119
Cheddar (Generic)	1 oz	114	30
Cheddar (Kraft)	1 oz	110	30
Cheddar (Land O Lakes)	1 oz	110	30
Cheddar (Tillamook)	1 oz	120	30
Cheddar, Low Sodium (Tillamook)	1 oz	120	30
Cheddar, Shredded (Weight Watchers)	1 oz	80	28
Cheddar, Shredded Low Sodium (Weight Watchers)	1 oz	80	28
Cheshire (Generic)	⅔ × 1 × 1″	110	29
Colby (Generic)	⅔ × 1 × 1″	112	27
Colby (Kraft)	1 oz	110	30
Colby (Land O Lakes)	1 oz	110	25
Cottage Cheese, 1% fat (Friendship)	½ cup (4 oz)	90	4.5
Cottage Cheese, 1% fat (Generic)	½ cup	81	5

FOOD	PORTION SIZE	CALORIES	CHOLESTEROL (Mg)
Cottage Cheese, 1% fat, Lactose Reduced (Friendship)	½ cup (4 oz)	90	4.5
Cottage Cheese, 1% fat, No Salt Added (Friendship)	½ cup (4 oz)	90	4.5
Cottage Cheese, 2% fat (Generic)	½ cup	102	9
Cottage Cheese, 2% fat (Land O Lakes)	½ cup	100	10
Cottage Cheese, 2% fat, Large Curd Pot Style (Friendship)	½ cup (4 oz)	100	9
Cottage Cheese, 4% fat, California Style (Friendship)	½ cup (4 oz)	120	17
Cottage Cheese, 4% fat, Pineapple (Friendship)	½ cup (4 oz)	140	17
Cottage cheese, creamed large curd (Generic)	½ cup	116	17
Cottage cheese, creamed small curd (Generic)	½ cup	108	16
Cottage cheese, creamed, w/ fruit added (Generic)	½ cup	140	12
Cottage cheese, dry curd not packed (Generic)	½ cup	62	5
Edam (Generic)	⅔ × 1 × 1"	101	25
Edam (Holland Farm)	1 oz	97	25
Edam (Land O Lakes)	1 oz	100	25
Farmer Cheese (Friendship)	½ cup (4 oz)	160	40
Farmer Cheese (Generic)	1 oz	102	26
Farmer Cheese (Holland Farm)	1 oz	102	26
Farmer Cheese, w/o Salt Added (Friendship)	½ cup (4 oz)	160	40
Feta (Generic)	¾ × 1 × 1"	75	25
Fontina (Frigo)	1 oz	110	33

FOOD	PORTION SIZE	CALORIES	CHOLESTEROL (Mg)
Fontina (Generic)	⅔ × 1 × 1″	110	33
Gouda (Generic)	1 oz	101	32
Gouda (Holland Farm)	1 oz	103	27
Gouda (Kraft)	1 oz	110	30
Gouda (Land O Lakes)	1 oz	100	30
Gruyere (Generic)	1 oz	117	31
Havarti, *Casino Brand* (Kraft)	1 oz	120	35
Hoop Cheese (Friendship)	½ cup (4 oz)	84	8
Italian Blend Cheese, Grated (Kraft)	1 oz	120	20
Jack-By, Monterey Jack & Colby Cheddar (Dutch Garden)	1 oz	102	27
Liederkranz (Generic)	1 oz	93	26
Limburger (Generic)	1 oz	93	26
Limburger (Mohawk Valley Brand)	1 oz	70	20
Limburger, *Little Gem Size* (Mohawk Valley Brand)	1 oz	90	25
Monterey Jack (Holland Farms)	1 oz	102	26
Monterey Jack (Kraft)	1 oz	110	30
Monterey Jack (Land O Lakes)	1 oz	110	20
Monterey Jack, w/Jalapeno Pepper (Kraft)	1 oz	110	30
Monterey Jack, w/Peppers, Mild (Kraft)	1 oz	110	30
Mozzarella (Generic)	1 oz	80	22
Mozzarella, *Casino Brand* (Kraft)	1 oz	90	25
Mozzarella, Lite (Polly-O)	1 oz	70	15
Mozzarella, Natural Sticks (Weight Watchers)	1 oz	70	29
Mozzarella, Part-Skim (Frigo)	1 oz	80	10

FOOD	PORTION SIZE	CALORIES	CHOLESTEROL (Mg)
Mozzarella, part-skim (Generic)	1 oz	80	15
Mozzarella, Part-Skim (Kraft)	1 oz	80	15
Mozzarella, Part-Skim (Land O Lakes)	1 oz	80	15
Mozzarella, Part-Skim (Polly-O)	1 oz	80	15
Mozzarella, Part-Skim w/ Jalapeno Pepper (Kraft)	1 oz	80	20
Mozzarella, Shredded (Weight Watchers)	1 oz	70	28
Mozzarella, Whole Milk (Frigo)	1 oz	90	15
Mozzarella, Whole Milk (Polly-O)	1 oz	90	20
Muenster (Generic)	1 slice	105	27
Muenster (Holland Farm)	1 oz	102	27
Muenster (Kraft)	1 oz	110	30
Muenster (Land O Lakes)	1 oz	100	25
Natural Sticks, Low Sodium (Weight Watchers)	1 oz	80	28
Neufchatel (Generic)	1 oz	74	22
Neufchatel (Kraft)	1 oz	80	25
Parmesan (Generic)	1 oz	111	19
Parmesan, grated (Frigo)	1 oz	130	25
Parmesan, grated (Generic)	1 Tbsp	23	4
Parmesan, grated (Kraft)	1 oz	130	30
Parmesan, loaf (Frigo)	1 oz	110	14
Parmesan, natural (Kraft)	1 oz	110	20
Parmesan, Zesty (Frigo)	1 oz	120	20
Parmesan & Romano, Grated (Frigo)	1 oz	130	29
Port du Salut (Generic)	1 oz	100	35
Provolone (Frigo)	1 oz	100	20
Provolone (Kraft)	1 oz	100	25
Provolone (Land O Lakes)	1 oz	100	20
Provolone, slice (Generic)	4⅝" diam × ⅛"	100	20

FOOD	PORTION SIZE	CALORIES	CHOLESTEROL (Mg)
Ricotta, *Lite* (Polly-O)	2 oz	80	15
Ricotta, Lowfat (Frigo)	1 oz	20	5
Ricotta, Part-Skim (Frigo)	1 oz	45	10
Ricotta, part-skim (Generic)	½ cup	170	38
Ricotta, Part-Skim (Polly-O)	2 oz	90	20
Ricotta, Whole Milk (Frigo)	1 oz	50	15
Ricotta, whole milk (Generic)	½ cup	214	63
Ricotta, Whole Milk (Polly-O)	2 oz	100	20
Romano, Grated (Frigo)	1 oz	130	35
Romano, Grated (Generic)	1 Tbsp	19	5
Romano, Grated (Kraft)	1 oz	130	30
Romano, Loaf (Frigo)	1 oz	110	30
Romano, Natural, *Casino Brand* (Kraft)	1 oz	100	30
Roquefort (Generic)	1 oz	105	26
Scamorze, Part-Skim (Kraft)	1 oz	80	15
String (Polly-O)	1 oz (1 stick)	90	15
Swiss (Generic)	1 oz	107	26
Swiss (Kraft)	1 oz	110	25
Swiss (Land O Lakes)	1 oz	110	25
Swiss (Sargento)	1 oz	107	26
Swiss, Aged (Kraft)	1 oz	110	25
Taco, Shredded Cheese (Frigo)	1 oz	110	30
Tilsit (Generic)	2×1×1"	97	29
Yogurt cheese (Home recipe)	1 oz	20	7

CHEESE, PROCESSED
(*see also* CHEESE, NATURAL; CHEESE DISHES; CREAM CHEESE)

FOOD	PORTION SIZE	CALORIES	CHOLESTEROL (Mg)
Ball, Sharp Cheddar w/ Almonds *Cracker Barrel Brand* (Kraft)	1 oz	90	15

FOOD	PORTION SIZE	CALORIES	CHOLESTEROL (Mg)
Food, American Cheese, Grated (Kraft)	1 oz	70	10
Food, American Flavored Pasteurized Process, *Harvest Moon Brand* (Kraft)	1 oz	70	15
Food, American Singles Pasteurized Process (Kraft)	1 oz	90	20
Food, Extra Sharp Cheddar Cold Pack, *Cracker Barrel Brand* (Kraft)	1 oz	90	20
Food, Jalapeno (Land O Lakes)	1 oz	90	20
Food, *La Chedda* (Land O Lakes)	1 oz	90	20
Food, Onion (Land O Lakes)	1 oz	90	15
Food, Pasteurized Process *Smokelle* (Kraft)	1 oz	100	20
Food, Pepperoni (Land O Lakes)	1 oz	90	20
Food, Port Wine Cheddar Cold Pack, *Cracker Barrel Brand* (Kraft)	1 oz	90	20
Food, Salami (Land O Lakes)	1 oz	100	20
Food, Sharp Cheddar Cold Pack, *Cracker Barrel Brand* (Kraft)	1 oz	90	20
Food, w/Bacon, Pasteurized Process (Kraft)	1 oz	90	20
Food, w/Garlic, Pasteurized Process (Kraft)	1 oz	90	20
Food, w/Real Bacon, Cold Pack *Cracker Barrel Brand* (Kraft)	1 oz	90	20
Imitation, American Flavored, Pasteurized Process *Golden Image* (Kraft)	1 oz	90	5

FOOD	PORTION SIZE	CALORIES	CHOLESTEROL (Mg)
Imitation, Cheddar (Frigo)	1 oz	70	none
Imitation, Cheddar, Mild *Golden Image* (Kraft)	1 oz	110	5
Imitation, Cheese Substitute, Skim Milk, *Smokey Flavor* (Count Down Fisher)	1 oz	34	1
Imitation, Colby, *Golden Image* (Kraft)	1 oz	110	5
Imitation, Low Cholesterol, *Lite-line* (Borden)	1 oz	90	5
Imitation, Mozzarella (Frigo)	1 oz	90	none
Imitation, Pastuerized, *Lite-line* (Borden)	1 oz	50	10
Loaf, American (Land O Lakes)	1 oz	110	25
Loaf, American/Swiss (Land O Lakes)	1 oz	100	25
Loaf, Pasteurized Process *Harvest Moon Brand* (Kraft)	1 oz	50	10
Loaf, American, Pasteurized Process *Deluxe* (Kraft)	1 oz	110	25
Loaf, Sharp, American, Pasteurized Process, *Old English* (Kraft)	1 oz	110	30
Log, Port Wine Cheddar, w/ Almonds, *Cracker Barrel Brand* (Kraft)	1 oz	90	15
Log, Sharp Cheddar w/ Almonds *Cracker Barrel Brand* (Kraft)	1 oz	90	15
Log, Smoky Cheddar w/ Almonds *Cracker Barrel Brand* (Kraft)	1 oz	90	15
Slices, American, Pasteurized Process, *Deluxe* (Kraft)	1 oz	110	25

FOOD	PORTION SIZE	CALORIES	CHOLESTEROL (Mg)
Slices, American Flavored Pasteurized Process, *Light N'Lively* (Kraft)	1 oz	70	15
Slices, Colored/white (Weight Watchers)	1 oz	45	8
Slices, Jalapeno, Pasteurized Process (Kraft)	1 oz	90	25
Slices, Low Sodium (Weight Watchers)	1 oz	50	8
Slices, Monterey Jack, Pasteurized Process (Kraft)	1 oz	90	25
Slices, Muenster Flavored Semisoft, Part-Skim (Naturally Slender)	1 oz	90	10
Slices, Pasteurized Process *Cheez 'N Bacon Singles* (Kraft)	1 oz	90	20
Slices, Pasteurized Process *Velveeta* (Kraft)	1 oz	90	20
Slices, Pimento, Pasteurized Process (Kraft)	1 oz	90	20
Slices, Pimento, Pasteurized Process *Deluxe* (Kraft)	1 oz	100	25
Slices, Swiss, Pasteurized Process *Deluxe* (Kraft)	1 oz	90	25
Slices, Sharp, Pasteurized Process (Kraft)	1 oz	100	25
Slices, Sharp, Pasteurized Process American, *Old English* (Kraft)	1 oz	110	30
Slices, Sharp Cheddar Flavored, Pasteurized Process, *Light N'Lively* (Kraft)	1 oz	70	15

FOOD	PORTION SIZE	CALORIES	CHOLESTEROL (Mg)
Slices, Swiss Flavor (Weight Watchers)	1 oz	50	8
Slices, Swiss, Pasteurized Process (Kraft)	1 oz	90	25
Slices, Swiss Flavored, Pasteurized Process, *Light N'Lively* (Kraft)	1 oz	70	15
Spread, American, Pasteurized Process (Kraft)	1 oz	80	20
Spread, Garlic Flavor, Pasteurized Process, *Squeez-A-Snak* (Kraft)	1 oz	90	20
Spread, *Golden Velvet* (Land O Lakes)	1 oz	80	70
Spread, Hickory Smoke Flavor, Pasteurized Process, *Squeez-A-Snak* (Kraft)	1 oz	80	20
Spread, Hot Mexican, Pasteurized Process, *Velveeta* (Kraft)	1 oz	80	20
Spread, Jalapeno, Pasteurized Process (Kraft)	1 oz	80	20
Spread, Jalapeno Pepper, Pasteurized Process (Kraft)	1 oz	70	15
Spread, Mild Mexican, Pasteurized Process, *Velveeta* (Kraft)	1 oz	80	20
Spread, Olives & Pimento, Pasteurized Process (Kraft)	1 oz	60	15
Spread, Pasteurized Process *Cheez Whiz* (Kraft)	1 oz	80	20
Spread, w/Jalapeno Peppers, Pasteurized Process, *Cheez Whiz* (Kraft)	1 oz	80	15

FOOD	PORTION SIZE	CALORIES	CHOLESTEROL (Mg)
Spread, Pasteurized Process, *Velveeta* (Kraft)	1 oz	80	20
Spread, Pimento, Pasteurized Process, *Velveeta* (Kraft)	1 oz	80	20
Spread, Pimento, Pasteurized Process, *Cheez Whiz* (Kraft)	1 oz	80	15
Spread, Pimento, Pasteurized Process (Kraft)	1 oz	70	15
Spread, Pineapple, Pasteurized Process (Kraft)	1 oz	70	15
Spread, Relish, Pasteurized Process (Kraft)	1 oz	70	15
Spread, Sharp, Pasteurized Process *Squeez-A-Snak* (Kraft)	1 oz	80	20
Spread, Sharp, Pasteurized Process *Old English* (Kraft)	1 oz	90	20
Spread, Sharp, Pasteurized Process *Velveeta* (Kraft)	1 oz	80	20
Spread, w/Bacon, Pasteurized Process (Kraft)	1 oz	80	20
Spread, w/Bacon, Pasteurized Process *Squeez-A-Snak* (Kraft)	1 oz	90	20
Spread, w/Garlic, Pasteurized Process (Kraft)	1 oz	80	15
Spread w/Pimento, Pasteurized Process *Squeez-A-Snak* (Kraft)	1 oz	90	20
Sticks, Colored/White Natural (Weight Watchers)	1 oz	80	28

FOOD	PORTION SIZE	CALORIES	CHOLESTEROL (Mg)

CHEESE DISHES

FOOD	PORTION SIZE	CALORIES	CHOLESTEROL (Mg)
Blintzes (Home recipe)	2	286	149
Fondue (Home recipe)	½ cup	303	62
Straws (Home recipe)	5×2×⅝″	266	82

CHICKEN

(see also CHICKEN DISHES; CHICKEN FRANKS; CHICKEN, FROZEN PREPARED; FROZEN DINNERS)

FOOD	PORTION SIZE	CALORIES	CHOLESTEROL (Mg)
Back, broiler/fryer, w/o skin; fried	1 piece	334	100
Back, broiler/fryer, w/o skin; roasted	1 piece	191	72
Back, broiler/fryer, w/o skin; stewed	1 piece	176	71
Back, broiler/fryer, w/skin; batter dipped, fried	1 piece	794	211
Back, broiler/fryer, w/skin; flour coated, fried	1 piece	477	128
Back, broiler/fryer, w/skin; roasted	1 piece	318	93
Back, broiler/fryer, w/skin; stewed	1 piece	315	95
Breast, broiler/fryer, w/skin; roasted	½ breast	193	82
Breast, broiler/fryer, w/o skin; roasted	½ breast	142	73
Breast, broiler/fryer, w/skin; stewed	½ breast	202	82
Breast, broiler/fryer, w/o skin; stewed	½ breast	143	73
Breast, broiler/fryer, w/skin; batter dipped, fried	½ breast	364	119

FOOD	PORTION SIZE	CALORIES	CHOLESTEROL (Mg)
Breast, broiler/fryer, w/skin; flour coated, fried	½ breast	218	87
Breast, broiler/fryer, w/o skin; fried	½ breast	161	78
Capons, meat w/skin; roasted	1 piece	195	73
Chicken Fat	1 Tbsp	126	12
Chicken roll (Generic)	3 slices 3" diam × ¼" thick	135	42
Dark meat, broiler/fryer, w/ skin; batter dipped, fried	2 pieces	242	78
Dark meat, broiler/fryer, w/ skin; roasted	2 pieces	215	77
Dark meat, broiler/fryer, w/ skin; stewed	2 pieces	198	70
Dark meat, broiler/fryer, w/o skin; fried, chopped	½ cup	167	67
Dark meat, broiler/fryer, w/o skin; roasted, chopped	½ cup	143	65
Dark meat, broiler/fryer, w/o skin; stewed, chopped	½ cup	134	62
Drumstick, broiler/fryer, w/skin; batter dipped, fried	1 piece	193	62
Drumstick, broiler/fryer, w/skin; flour coated, fried	1 piece	120	44
Drumstick, broiler/fryer, w/skin; roasted	1 piece	112	47
Drumstick, broiler/fryer, w/skin; stewed	1 piece	116	47
Drumstick, broiler/fryer, w/o skin; fried	1 piece	82	39
Drumstick, broiler/fryer, w/o skin; roasted	1 piece	76	41

FOOD	PORTION SIZE	CALORIES	CHOLESTEROL (Mg)
Drumstick, broiler, fryer, w/o skin; stewed	1 piece	78	40
Leg, broiler/fryer, w/skin; batter dipped, fried	1 piece	431	142
Leg, broiler/fryer, w/skin; flour coated, fried	1 piece	284	105
Leg, broiler/fryer, w/skin; roasted	1 piece	264	105
Leg, broiler/fryer, w/skin; stewed	1 piece	275	105
Leg, broiler/fryer, w/o skin; fried	1 piece	196	93
Leg, broiler/fryer, w/o skin; roasted	1 piece	181	89
Leg, broiler/fryer, w/o skin; stewed	1 piece	187	90
Light & dark meat, broiler/fryer, w/skin; batter dipped, fried	½ bird	1347	405
Light & dark meat, broiler/fryer, w/skin; flour coated, fried	½ bird	845	283
Light & dark meat, broiler/fryer, w/skin; roasted	½ bird	715	263
Light & dark meat, broiler/fryer, w/skin; stewed	½ bird	731	261
Light & dark meat, broiler/fryer, w/o skin; fried, chopped	½ bird	153	66
Light & dark meat, broiler/fryer, w/o skin; roasted, chopped	½ bird	133	62

FOOD	PORTION SIZE	CALORIES	CHOLESTEROL (Mg)
Light & dark meat, broiler/ fryer, w/o skin; stewed, chopped	½ cup	124	58
Light meat, broiler/fryer, w/ skin; batter dipped, fried	1 piece	235	71
Light meat, broiler/fryer, w/ skin; flour coated, fried	1 piece	209	74
Light meat, broiler/fryer, w/ skin; roasted	1 piece	189	71
Light meat, broiler/fryer, w/ skin; stewed	1 piece	171	63
Light meat, broiler/fryer, w/o skin; fried, chopped	½ cup	134	63
Light meat, broiler/fryer, w/o skin; roasted, chopped	½ cup	121	59
Light meat, broiler/fryer, w/o skin; stewed, chopped	½ cup	111	54
Neck, broiler/fryer, w/skin; batter dipped; fried	1 piece	172	47
Neck, broiler/fryer, w/skin; flour coated; fried	1 piece	120	34
Neck, broiler/fryer, w/skin; fried	1 piece	50	23
Neck, broiler/fryer, w/skin; stewed	1 piece (1⅓ oz)	94	27
Neck, broiler/fryer, w/skin; stewed	1 piece (½ oz)	32	14
Roaster, dark meat w/o skin; roasted, chopped	½ cup	125	52
Roaster, light & dark meat, w/o skin; roasted, chopped	½ cup	117	52
Roaster, light meat w/o skin; roasted chopped	½ cup	107	52
Shake 'n Bake, Oven Fry Seasoning, Coating Mix (General Foods)	1 Tbsp	20	none

FOOD	PORTION SIZE	CALORIES	CHOLESTEROL (Mg)
Skin; fried	1 oz	112	21
Skin; roasted	1 oz	129	24
Skin; stewed	1 oz	103	18
Stewing chicken, dark meat w/o skin; stewed, chopped	½ cup	181	66
Stewing chicken, light & dark, w/o skin; stewed, chopped	½ cup	166	58
Stewing chicken, light meat w/o skin; stewed, chopped	½ cup	149	49
Thigh, broiler/fryer, w/skin; batter dipped, fried	1 piece	238	80
Thigh, broiler/fryer, w/skin; flour coated, fried	1 piece	162	60
Thigh, broiler/fryer, w/skin; roasted	1 piece	153	58
Thigh, broiler/fryer, w/skin; stewed	1 piece	158	57
Thigh, broiler/fryer, w/o skin; fried	1 piece	113	53
Thigh, broiler/fryer, w/o skin; roasted	1 piece	109	49
Thigh, broiler/fryer, w/o skin; stewed	1 piece	107	49
Wing, broiler/fryer, w/skin; batter dipped, fried	1 piece	159	39
Wing, broiler/fryer, w/skin; flour coated, fried	1 piece	103	26
Wing, broiler/fryer, w/skin; roasted	1 piece	99	29
Wing, broiler/fryer, w/skin; stewed	1 piece	100	28
Wing, broiler/fryer, w/o skin; fried	1 piece	42	17
Wing, broiler/fryer, w/o skin; roasted	1 piece	43	18

FOOD	PORTION SIZE	CALORIES	CHOLESTEROL (Mg)
Wing, broiler/fryer, w/o skin; stewed	1 piece	43	18

CHICKEN DISHES
(*see also* CHICKEN; CHICKEN, FROZEN PREPARED; FROZEN DINNERS)

FOOD	PORTION SIZE	CALORIES	CHOLESTEROL (Mg)
A la king, creamed (Home recipe)	¾ cup	234	76
Cacciatore (Home recipe)	¾ cup	394	99
Casserole (Home recipe)	¾ cup	198	39
Dumplings & chicken (Home recipe)	¾ cup	256	109
Noodles & chicken (Home recipe)	¾ cup	191	43
Potpie (Home recipe)	1	706	118
Teriyaki (Home recipe)	¾ cup	399	92

CHICKEN, FROZEN PREPARED
(*see also* CHICKEN, CHICKEN DISHES, FROZEN DINNERS)

FOOD	PORTION SIZE	CALORIES	CHOLESTEROL (Mg)
Batter Dipped, Breasts (Weaver)	3 oz	255	72
Batter Dipped, Drum & Thighs (Weaver)	3 oz	255	76
Batter Dipped, Wings (Weaver)	3 oz	290	67
Chicken Roll (Weaver)	3 oz	174	37
Croquettes (Weaver)	3 oz	274	38
Dutch Frye, Breasts (Weaver)	3 oz	246	72
Dutch Frye, Drum & Thighs (Weaver)	3 oz	255	76

FOOD	PORTION SIZE	CALORIES	CHOLESTEROL (Mg)
Dutch Frye, Wings (Weaver)	3 oz	272	67
Mini-Drums, Crispy (Weaver)	3 oz	201	51
Nuggets (Weaver)	3 oz	226	74
Rondelets, Cheese (Weaver)	3 oz	220	33
Rondelets, Home Style (Weaver)	3 oz	200	46
Rondelets, Italian (Weaver)	3 oz	215	44
Rondelets, Original (Weaver)	3 oz	200	46
Thigh Fillet Strips (Weaver)	3 oz	262	81

CHILI

Vegetarian (Worthington)	½ cup	190	none
With beans (Home recipe)	½ cup	144	22

CHIPS & SNACKS

Chips, Corn, *Fritos*	1 oz	155	tr
Chips, Corn, Barbeque Flavor *Fritos*	1 oz	151	none
Chips, Potato *Lay's*	1 oz	153	tr
Chips, Potato, *Muchos*	1 oz	154	none
Chips, Potato, *Pringles*	1 oz	171	none
Chips, Potato, *Ruffles*	1 oz	151	tr
Chips, Potato, Bacon & Sour Cream Flavor, *Ruffles*	1 oz	152	1
Chips, Potato, Barbeque Flavor, *Lay's*	1 oz	149	tr
Chips, Potato, Barbeque Flavor, *Ruffles*	1 oz	147	tr
Chips, Potato, Cheese Flavor, *Lay's*	1 oz	153	1

FOOD	PORTION SIZE	CALORIES	CHOLESTEROL (Mg)
Chips, Potato, Cheese Flavor, *Ruffles*	1 oz	154	1
Chips, Potato, Light Style, *Pringles*	1 oz	144	none
Chips, Potato, No Salt Added, *Lay's*	1 oz	156	none
Chips, Potato, Sour Cream & Onion, *Lay's*	1 oz	153	1
Chips, Potato, Sour Cream & Onion *Ruffles*	1 oz	153	1
Chips, Tortilla, *Doritos*	1 oz	139	none
Chips, Tortilla, Cheese Flavor *Doritos*	1 oz	144	tr
Chips, Tortilla, Extra Crispy, *Doritos*	1 oz	145	tr
Chips, Tortilla, Extra Crispy, Cheese Flavor, *Doritos*	1 oz	148	1
Chips, Tortilla, Nacho Cheese, *Doritos*	1 oz	140	none
Chips, Tortilla, Round, *Tostitos*	1 oz	145	tr
Chips, Tortilla, Round, Cheese Flavor, *Tostitos*	1 oz	148	1
Chips, Tortilla, Taco Flavor, *Doritos*	1 oz	139	none
Cornuts	1 oz	110	none
Funyuns	1 oz	140	tr
Pretzels, *Twists* (Rold Gold)	1 oz	112	none
Pretzels, *Quinlan*	1 oz	110	1
Pretzels, 100% Whole Wheat (Barbaras)	2	120	none
Snack Cracker, Cheddar, *American Heritage* (Sunshine)	5 crackers	80	20

FOOD	PORTION SIZE	CALORIES	CHOLESTEROL (Mg)
Snack Crackers, Cheez 'n Crackers *Handi-Snacks* (Kraft)	1 pkg	130	15
Snack Crackers, Peanut Butter 'n *Handi-Snacks* (Kraft)	1 pkg	190	none
Snacks, Cheese Puffs, *Cheetos*	1 oz	159	tr
Snacks, Cheese Puffs w/Bacon Flavor, *Cheetos*	1 oz	159	tr
Snacks, Cheese Snacks, *Cheetos*	1 oz	158	1
Snacks, French Fried Onions (Durkee)	2.8 oz can	468	none
Snacks, Pork Rinds, *Frito-Lay*	1 oz	151	24
Snacks, Puffed Balls, *Cheetos*	1 oz	161	1

CHINESE FOOD
(*see also* RICE)

FOOD	PORTION SIZE	CALORIES	CHOLESTEROL (Mg)
Chop suey, w/meat, canned (Generic)	1 cup	144	21
Chop suey, w/pork (Home recipe)	1 cup	375	62
Chow mein, chicken, canned (Generic)	1 cup	95	8
Chow mein, chicken (Home recipe)	1 cup	255	78
Chow mein, pork (Home recipe)	1 cup	425	89
Chow mein, shrimp (Home recipe)	1 cup	221	55

FOOD	PORTION SIZE	CALORIES	CHOLESTEROL (Mg)

CHITTERLINGS
(*see* PORK)

CHOCOLATE/COCOA
(*see also* CANDY, MILK, MILK DRINKS, MILK FLAVORINGS)

FOOD	PORTION SIZE	CALORIES	CHOLESTEROL (Mg)
Baking, Chocolate, Unsweetened (Hershey)	1 oz sq	188	4
Chips, chocolate flavored (Generic)	¼ cup	195	tr
Chips, milk chocolate (Generic)	¼ cup	218	7
Choco-Bake (Nestle)	1 oz	170	none
Chunks Chocolate (Saco)	6 chunks	80	none
Cocoa (Hershey)	3½ oz	410	4
Cocoa, Premium Baking (Saco)	1 Tbsp	15	none
Mix, carob flavor (Generic)	3 tsp	45	none
Mix, carob flavor; as prep w/ whole milk (Generic)	1 cup	195	33
Mix, chocolate flavor, powder (Generic)	2–3 heaping tsp	75	none
Mix, Instant (Hershey)	3½ oz	360	none
Syrup, chocolate (Generic)	2 Tbsp	82	none
Syrup, chocolate; as prep w/ whole milk (Generic)	1 cup	232	33
Syrup, Chocolate Flavored (Hershey)	3½ oz	260	none

COCONUT

FOOD	PORTION SIZE	CALORIES	CHOLESTEROL (Mg)
Cream, canned (Generic)	½ cup	284	none
Dry, sweetened, chopped (Generic)	¼ cup	85	none

FOOD	PORTION SIZE	CALORIES	CHOLESTEROL (Mg)
Fresh	¼ cup	84	none
Milk (Generic)	½ cup	26	none
Shredded (Bakers)	⅓ cup	140	none

COFFEE/TEA

FOOD	PORTION SIZE	CALORIES	CHOLESTEROL (Mg)
Coffee, brewed or instant or decaf (Generic)	8 oz	0	none
Coffee, *International Coffees, Suisse Mocha* (General Foods)	2 tsp	55	none
Coffee substitute, cereal grain powder (Generic)	1 tsp	9	none
Tea; brewed (Generic)	8 oz.	0	none
Tea, herb; brewed (Generic)	8 oz	0	none
Tea, instant, lemon flavor, unsweetened powder (Generic)	1 tsp	4	none
Tea, unsweetened powder (Generic)	1 tsp	2	none

COFFEE WHITENERS

FOOD	PORTION SIZE	CALORIES	CHOLESTEROL (Mg)
Coffee-Mate (Carnation)	1 tsp	11	tr
Creamora (Borden)	1 tsp	12	none

COLD CUTS
(*see* LUNCHEON MEATS/COLD CUTS)

FOOD	PORTION SIZE	CALORIES	CHOLESTEROL (Mg)

COLE SLAW
(*see* SALADS)

COOKIES
(*see also* CAKE, DOUGHNUTS, PIE, QUICHE)

FOOD	PORTION SIZE	CALORIES	CHOLESTEROL (Mg)
Animal Crackers (Sunshine)	14 pieces	120	none
Brownie w/nuts (Home recipe)	1¾" sq × ⅞"	97	15
Butter Flavored (Sunshine)	4 cookies	120	5
Butter, Christmas, rolled sugar (Home recipe)	2½" diam	50	5
Chocolate chip (Home recipe)	2½" diam	59	5
Chocolate Fudge Sandwich (Sunshine)	2 cookies	150	none
Chocolate oatmeal (Generic)	2" diam	66	5
Cinnamon Graham (Sunshine)	4 cookies	70	none
Cup Custard, Cookie (Sunshine)	2 cookies	130	5
Fig Bar (Keebler)	1 cookie	71	12
Fig Bar (Sunshine)	2 cookies	90	none
Fortune Cookie (Generic)	1 cookie	66	8
Ginger snaps (Generic)	2" diam	30	2
Ginger Snaps (Sunshine)	5 cookies	100	none
Grahamy Bears (Sunshine)	9 cookies	130	none
Honey Graham (Sunshine)	4 cookies	60	none
Lemon bar (Home recipe)	2 × 2"	110	37
Lemon Coolers (Sunshine)	5 cookies	140	none
Lorna Doone Shortbread (R.J. Reynolds)	3 cookies	140	10
Macaroon (Generic)	2½" diam	54	none
Mallopuffs (Sunshine)	2 cookies	140	none
Molasses cookie (Home recipe)	3⅝" diam	138	25

FOOD	PORTION SIZE	CALORIES	CHOLESTEROL (Mg)
Oatmeal Peanut Sandwich (Sunshine)	2 cookies	140	none
Oatmeal w/raisin (Home recipe)	2⅝" diam	54	5
Peanut butter cookie (Home recipe)	2" diam	61	5
Peanut Butter Wafers (Sunshine)	3 cookies	120	none
Pecan Sandies (Keebler)	1 cookie	85	none
Pumpkin bar (Home recipe)	2 × 2"	151	25
Raisin Biscuits, *Golden Fruits* (Sunshine)	2 cookies	150	none
Raspberry bar (Home recipe)	1 cookie	76	6
Sprinkles (Sunshine)	2 cookies	130	none
Sugar cookie (Home recipe)	2¼" diam	36	8
Toy Cookies (Sunshine)	10 cookies	120	none
Vanilla Wafers (Sunshine)	6 wafers	130	5

CORN CHIPS
(*see* CHIPS & SNACKS)

CORN MEAL

Enriched Yellow, *Aunt Jemima* (Quaker)	1 cup	544	none

CORN STARCH

ARGO (Best Foods)	1 Tbsp	30	none

FOOD	PORTION SIZE	CALORIES	CHOLESTEROL (Mg)

CORN
(*see* VEGETABLES)

CRACKERS

FOOD	PORTION SIZE	CALORIES	CHOLESTEROL (Mg)
Cheddar Snack Crackers *American Heritage,* (Sunshine)	5 crackers	80	5
Cheez-It, Low Salt (Sunshine)	12 crackers	70	none
Crispbread, Lite, *Wasa*	3 pieces (1 oz)	90	none
Handi-Snacks Cheez 'n Crackers (Kraft)	1 pkg	130	15
Handi-Snacks Peanut Butter 'n Cheez Crackers (Kraft)	1 pkg	190	none
Matzo, Daily Thin Tea (Manischewitz)	1 piece (.91 oz)	103	none
Matzo, Egg N'Onion (Manischewitz)	1 piece (1 oz)	112	15
Matzo, Miniatures (Manischewitz)	15 crackers	90	none
Matzo, Passover (Manischewitz)	1 piece	129	none
Matzo, Passover Egg (Manischewitz)	1 piece	132	25
Matzo, Passover Egg, Cracker Size (Manischewitz)	10 crackers	108	20
Matzo, Thins Dietetic (Manischewitz)	1 piece (.83 oz)	91	none
Matzo, Unsalted (Manischewitz)	1 piece (1 oz)	110	none
Matzo, Wheat, Cracker Size (Manischewitz)	10 crackers	90	none

FOOD	PORTION SIZE	CALORIES	CHOLESTEROL (Mg)
Matzo, Whole Wheat W/Bran (Manischewitz)	1 piece	110	none
Oyster & Soup Crackers (Sunshine)	16 crackers	60	none
Ritz (Nabisco)	9 crackers (1 oz)	150	<10
Rye w/Cheese (Frito Lay)	1.5 oz	205	4
Saltine *Premium* (Nabisco)	10 crackers (1 oz)	120	<10
Sesame (Pepperidge Farm)	4 crackers	80	none
Tams, Garlic (Manischewitz)	10 crackers	153	none
Tams, Onion (Manischewitz)	10 crackers	150	none
Tams, Tam, No Salt (Manischewitz)	5 crackers	70	none
Tams, Wheat (Manischewitz)	10 crackers	150	none
Toast crackers w/peanut butter (Generic)	1.5 oz	212	tr
Town House (Keebler)	9 crackers	157	tr
Triscuit Wafers	6 wafers (1 oz)	140	none
Uneeda Biscuits	6 biscuits (1 oz)	130	none
Waldorf, low salt (Keebler)	9 crackers	130	none
Wheat Crackers w/Cheese (Frito Lay)	1.5 oz	212	4
Wheat Thins (Nabisco)	16 crackers (1 oz)	130	none
W/Cheese (Frito Lay)	1.5 oz	198	5
Zwieback (Generic)	4 pieces	119	6

FOOD	PORTION SIZE	CALORIES	CHOLESTEROL (Mg)

CREAM
(see also SOUR CREAM, WHIPPED TOPPINGS)

FOOD	PORTION SIZE	CALORIES	CHOLESTEROL (Mg)
Half & half (Generic)	1 Tbsp	20	6
Half & Half (Land O Lakes)	1 Tbsp	20	5
Heavy whipping (Generic)	1 Tbsp	51	20
Heavy Whipping, Gourmet (Land O Lakes)	1 Tbsp	60	20
Heavy whipping, whipped (Generic)	¼ cup	103	41
Light, coffee or table (Generic)	1 Tbsp	29	10
Light whipping (Generic)	1 Tbsp	44	17
Medium, 25% fat (Generic)	1 Tbsp	36	13
Real Cream Topping (Kraft)	¼ cup	25	10
Whipped cream topping, pressurized (Generic)	¼ cup	39	11
Whipping Cream (Land O Lakes)	1 Tbsp	45	15

CREAM CHEESE

FOOD	PORTION SIZE	CALORIES	CHOLESTEROL (Mg)
Regular (Generic)	1 oz	99	31
Regular, *Philadelphia Brand* (Kraft)	1 oz	100	30
Regular, With Chives, *Philadelphia Brand* (Kraft)	1 oz	90	30
Regular, With Pimentos *Philadelphia Brand* (Kraft)	1 oz	90	30
Soft (Friendship)	1 oz	103	31
Soft *Philadelphia Brand* (Kraft)	1 oz	100	30
Soft, With Chives and Onions, *Philadelphia Brand* (Kraft)	1 oz	100	30
Soft, With Peaches, *Philadelphia Brand* (Kraft)	1 oz	90	25

FOOD	PORTION SIZE	CALORIES	CHOLESTEROL (Mg)
Soft, With Pineapple, *Philadelphia Brand* (Kraft)	1 oz	90	25
Soft, With Strawberries, *Philadelphia Brand* (Kraft)	1 oz	90	25
Whipped *Philadelphia Brand* (Kraft)	1 oz	100	30
Whipped With Bacon and Horseradish *Philadelphia Brand* (Kraft)	1 oz	90	20
Whipped, With Blue Cheese, *Philadelphia Brand* (Kraft)	1 oz	100	25
Whipped, With Chives, *Philadelphia Brand* (Kraft)	1 oz	90	25
Whipped, With Onions *Philadelphia Brand* (Kraft)	1 oz	90	20
Whipped, With Pimentos *Philadelphia Brand* (Kraft)	1 oz	90	20
Whipped, With Smoked Salmon, *Philadelphia Brand* (Kraft)	1 oz	100	25

CREPES
(*see also* FRENCH TOAST, PANCAKES/HOT CAKES, WAFFLES)

FOOD	PORTION SIZE	CALORIES	CHOLESTEROL (Mg)
Apple, frzn (Mrs. Smith's)	1 crepe	195	15
Chicken Continental, frzn (Mrs. Smith's)	2 crepes	320	65
Chicken Maison, frzn (Mrs. Smith's)	2 crepes	350	70
Ham & Vegetables, frzn (Mrs. Smith's)	2 crepes	305	70
Shrimp, frzn (Mrs. Smith's)	2 crepes	305	105
Strawberry, frzn (Mrs. Smith's)	1 crepe	150	15

FOOD	PORTION SIZE	CALORIES	CHOLESTEROL (Mg)

CROUTONS
(*see* BREAD & ROLLS)

CUP-A-SOUP
(*see* SOUPS, DRY)

CUSTARD

FOOD	PORTION SIZE	CALORIES	CHOLESTEROL (Mg)
Baked (Home recipe)	½ cup	152	139
Mix; as prep (Generic)	½ cup	161	80
Reduced Calorie; made w/skim milk (Delmark)	½ cup	97	6

DAIRY QUEEN

ICE CREAM

FOOD	PORTION SIZE	CALORIES	CHOLESTEROL (Mg)
Banana Split	1	540	30
Buster Bar	1	460	10
Cone, lg	1	340	25
Cone, reg	1	240	15
Cone, sm	1	140	10
Dilly Bar	1	210	10
Dipped cone, lg	1	510	30
Dipped cone, reg	1	340	20
Dipped cone, sm	1	190	10
Double Delight	1	490	25
Float	1	410	20
Fudge Nut Bar	1	406	10
Freeze	1	500	30

FOOD	PORTION SIZE	CALORIES	CHOLESTEROL (Mg)
Heath Blizzard	1	800	65
Hot Fudge Brownie Delight	1	600	20
Malt, lg	1	1060	70
Malt, reg	1	760	50
Malt, sm	1	520	35
Mr. Misty, lg	1	340	none
Mr. Misty, reg	1	250	none
Mr. Misty, sm	1	190	none
Mr. Misty Float	1	390	20
Mr. Misty Freeze	1	500	30
Mr. Misty Kiss	1	70	none
Parfait	1	430	30
Peanut Buster Parfait	1	740	30
Shake, lg	1	990	70
Shake, reg	1	710	50
Shake, sm	1	490	35
Strawberry Shortcake	1	540	25
Sundae, lg	1	440	30
Sundae, reg	1	310	20
Sundae, sm	1	190	10

FOOD SELECTIONS

Chicken Sandwich	1	670	75
Double Hamburger	1	530	85
Double w/Cheese	1	650	95
DQ Sandwich	1	140	5
Fish Filet Sandwich	1	400	50
Fish Filet Sandwich w/Cheese	1	440	60
French Fries, lg	1	320	15
French Fries, sm	1	200	10
Hot Dog	1	280	45
Hot Dog w/Cheese	1	330	55
Hot Dog w/Chili	1	320	55

FOOD	PORTION SIZE	CALORIES	CHOLESTEROL (Mg)
Onion Rings	1	280	15
Single Hamburger	1	360	45
Single w/Cheese	1	410	50
Super Hot Dog	1	520	80
Super Hot Dog w/Cheese	1	580	100
Super Hot Dog w/Chili	1	570	100
Triple Hamburger	1	710	135
Triple w/Cheese	1	820	145

DINNERS
(*see* FROZEN DINNERS, NOODLES & PASTA)

DIPS
(*see also* GRAVY; SALAD DRESSINGS; SAUCES; SOUPS, DRY)
All of the following dips are ready-to-serve

FOOD	PORTION SIZE	CALORIES	CHOLESTEROL (Mg)
Avocado, Guacamole (Kraft)	2 Tbsp	50	none
Bacon & Horseradish (Kraft)	2 Tbsp	60	none
Bacon & Horseradish, *Premium* (Kraft)	1 oz	50	10
Blue Cheese, *Premium* (Kraft)	1 oz	45	20
Buttermilk (Kraft)	2 Tbsp	70	none
Buttermilk, *Lean Cream* (Land O Lakes)	2 Tbsp	40	7
Clam (Kraft)	2 Tbsp	60	10
Clam, *Premium* (Kraft)	1 oz	45	20
Cucumber, Creamy, *Premium* (Kraft)	1 oz	50	10
Dill, *Lean Cream* (Land O Lakes)	2 Tbsp	40	7

FOOD	PORTION SIZE	CALORIES	CHOLESTEROL (Mg)
French Onion (Kraft)	2 Tbsp	60	none
French Onion, *Lean Cream* (Land O Lakes)	2 Tbsp	40	7
French Onion, *Premium* (Kraft)	1 oz	45	10
Garlic (Kraft)	2 Tbsp	60	none
Green Onion (Kraft)	2 Tbsp	60	none
Jalapeno Pepper (Kraft)	2 Tbsp	50	none
Jalapeno Pepper, *Premium* (Kraft)	1 oz	60	15
Jalapeno, *Lean Cream* (Land O Lakes)	2 Tbsp	40	7
Nacho Cheese, *Premium* (Kraft)	1 oz	50	10
Onion, Creamy, *Premium* (Kraft)	1 oz	45	10
Onion & Garlic, *Lean Cream* (Land o'Lakes)	2 Tbsp	40	7

DOMINO'S PIZZA
(*see also* PIZZA)
Portion based on 2 slices of an 8-slice small pizza

FOOD	PORTION SIZE	CALORIES	CHOLESTEROL (Mg)
Double Cheese	2 slices	480	35
Double Cheese, Pepperoni	2 slices	453	46
Ground Beef	2 slices	361	30
Ground Beef, Pepperoni	2 slices	431	46
Mushroom, Sausage	2 slices	365	28
Pepperoni	2 slices	384	34
Pepperoni, Mushroom	2 slices	388	34
Pepperoni, Sausage	2 slices	431	44
Plain Cheese	2 slices	314	17
Sausage	2 slices	360	28

FOOD	PORTION SIZE	CALORIES	CHOLESTEROL (Mg)
Portion based on 2 slices of an 8-slice 10″ pizza			
Double Cheese	2 slices	284	24
Double Cheese, Pepperoni	2 slices	331	35
Ground Beef	2 slices	250	21
Ground Beef, Pepperoni	2 slices	297	32
Mushroom, Sausage	2 slices	248	18
Pepperoni	2 slices	265	23
Pepperoni, Mushroom	2 slices	267	23
Pepperoni, Sausage	2 slices	293	29
Plain Cheese	2 slices	218	12
Sausage	2 slices	246	18
Portion based on 2 slices of a 12-slice 14″ pizza			
Double Cheese	2 slices	365	31
Double Cheese, Pepperoni	2 slices	427	45
Ground Beef	2 slices	321	26
Ground Beef, Pepperoni	2 slices	382	40
Mushroom Sausage	2 slices	322	24
Pepperoni	2 slices	343	29
Pepperoni, Mushroom	2 slices	346	29
Pepperoni, Sausage	2 slices	380	38
Plain Cheese	2 slices	281	15
Sausage	2 slices	318	24
Portion based on 2 slices of a 12-slice large pizza			
Double Cheese	2 slices	700	42
Double Cheese Pepperoni	2 slices	778	60
Ground Beef	2 slices	527	34
Ground Beef, Pepperoni	2 slices	605	52
Mushroom Sausage	2 slices	532	33
Pepperoni	2 slices	556	39
Pepperoni Mushroom	2 slices	560	39
Pepperoni, Sausage	2 slices	606	51

FOOD	PORTION SIZE	CALORIES	CHOLESTEROL (Mg)
Plain Cheese	2 slices	478	21
Sausage	2 slices	528	33

DOUGHNUTS
(*see also* CAKE, COOKIES, PIE, QUICHE)

Cake, Doughnut (Hostess)	1	115	7
Cinnamon (Hostess)	1	109	6
Chocolate Covered (Hostess)	1	129	4
Krunch (Hostess)	1	101	4
Old Fashioned (Hostess)	1	172	10
Powdered Sugar (Hostess)	1	112	7
Jelly filled, raised (Home recipe)	1	226	21
Yeast, raised (Home recipe)	1	174	17

DUCK

W/skin; roasted	½ duck	1287	320
W/o skin; roasted	½ duck	445	198

DUMPLING

Apple (Home recipe)	1	566	19
Pear (Home recipe)	1	540	41

EGGS

Creamed (Home recipe)	½ cup	231	310
Deviled (Home recipe)	2 halves	145	280

FOOD	PORTION SIZE	CALORIES	CHOLESTEROL (Mg)
Dry, plain (Generic)	1 cup	507	1615
Dry, stabilized (Generic)	1 cup	523	1714
Egg foo young (Home recipe)	1 avg	150	250
Fried in butter	1 lg	83	246
Hard cooked	1 lg	79	274
Low Cholesterol Egg (Environmental Systems)	1 extra lg	60	195
Omelet; as prep w/two eggs, 1 Tbsp butter, 2 Tbsp whole milk (Home recipe)	1 serving	276	582
Poached	1 lg	79	273
Raw	1 lg	79	279
Salad (Home recipe)	½ cup	307	562
Scrambled; as prep w/butter & whole milk	½ cup	163	427
Scrambled Eggs (McDonald's)	1 portion	180	514
Scrambled Eggs Breakfast (Jack in the Box)	1 portion	719	260
Scrambled Egg Platter (Burger King)	1 portion	468	370
White only	1 lg	14	none
Yolk only	1 lg	68	247

EGG SUBSTITUTE

FOOD	PORTION SIZE	CALORIES	CHOLESTEROL (Mg)
Egg Beaters, frzn (Fleischmann's)	¼ cup	40	none
Eggstra, as prep (Tillie Lewis)	1 serving	43	58
Frozen, made w/egg white & corn oil (Generic)	¼ cup	96	1
Powder (Generic)	1 oz	126	162

FOOD	PORTION SIZE	CALORIES	CHOLESTEROL (Mg)

FAST FOODS
(*see individual names*)

FATS
(*see also* BUTTER, MARGARINE, MAYONNAISE, OILS)

FOOD	PORTION SIZE	CALORIES	CHOLESTEROL (Mg)
Beef tallow, suet	1 Tbsp	116	14
Chicken fat	1 Tbsp	115	11
Crisco	1 Tbsp	106	none
Duck fat	1 Tbsp	115	13
Goose fat	1 Tbsp	115	13
Mutton tallow	1 Tbsp	116	13
Pork fat, lard	1 Tbsp	116	12
Turkey fat	1 Tbsp	115	13

FISH

FOOD	PORTION SIZE	CALORIES	CHOLESTEROL (Mg)
Caviar, sturgeon granular	1 Tbsp	42	48
Chub	3½ oz raw	145	50
Clam, hard or soft shell	1 med raw	13	8
Cod, dried, salted	3½ oz	130	82
Cod, fillet; broiled w/2 tsp butter	1 med	119	54
Cod, fillet; cooked	1 med	84	32
Cod, *Today's Catch* (Van de Kamp's)	4 oz	88	24
Crab leg; steamed in shell	1	40	43
Crab, blue hard shell; steamed whole	1	20	21
Crab; deviled	½ cup	182	125
Crab, Dungeness; steamed whole	1	64	68

FOOD	PORTION SIZE	CALORIES	CHOLESTEROL (Mg)
Crab, Imperial (Home recipe)	½ cup	162	154
Crab; steamed	3½ oz	93	100
Crab; stuffed (Home recipe)	¾ cup	129	123
Crabmeat; steamed pieces	½ cup	72	77
Crabmeat; steamed flaked	½ cup	58	63
Crabmeat, white or king, canned	½ cup	68	68
Eel, smoked	1¾ oz	165	35
Fish stick, frzn; breaded, cooked	3 sticks	200	80
Flounder, fillet; baked w/butter	1 fillet	113	28
Flounder, fillet; cooked	1 fillet	78	28
Flounder, *Today's Catch* (Van de Kamp's)	4 oz	80	54
Haddock, fillet; breaded, fried	1 med	181	66
Haddock, fillet; fried	1 med	71	47
Haddock, *Today's Catch* (Van de Kamp's)	4 oz	88	64
Halibut fillet; broiled w/butter	1 med	214	63
Halibut fillet; cooked	1 med	163	63
Halibut steak; broiled w/butter	1 med	144	42
Herring, Atlantic	3½ oz raw	176	85
Herring, canned	3 oz	156	73
Herring, pickled pieces	½ oz	33	13
Herring, pickled whole	1 herring 7" long	112	43
Herring, smoked kippered, filleted	1 med	84	34
Herring, smoked kippered, filleted	1 sm	42	17
Herring w/tomato sauce, canned	1 herring 7" long	97	53
Lobster; cooked, cubed	½ cup	69	62
Lobster Newburg (Home recipe)	1 cup	485	455

FOOD	PORTION SIZE	CALORIES	CHOLESTEROL (Mg)
Lobster tail; cooked	1 medium	99	88
Lobster whole; cooked	1 medium	107	96
Lox, smoked salmon	1 piece	35	15
Mackerel, Atlantic	3½ oz raw	191	95
Mussels, Pacific, canned	3½ oz	114	150
Oysters, canned	⅓ cup	61	36
Perch, *Today's Catch* (Van de Kamp's)	4 oz	128	64
Pollock, Fillet, *Today's Catch* (Van de Kamp's)	4 oz	128	64
Salmon cake (Home recipe)	3" cake	241	104
Salmon casserole (Home recipe)	¾ cup	416	91
Salmon, red sockeye, canned (Generic)	½ cup	188	38
Salmon, Pink, canned (Bumble Bee)	3.5 oz	160	65
Salmon, Red Sockeye, canned (Bumble Bee)	½ cup	188·	40
Salmon rice loaf (Home recipe)	5 oz	299	133
Salmon, Skinless-Boneless Chunk Pink, canned (Bumble Bee)	3.5 oz	130	65
Salmon, smoked	1 piece	35	15
Sardines, Atlantic, in oil, canned	1 med	24	17
Sardines, Pacific, in oil, canned	3½ oz	380	140
Sardines, Pacific, w/mustard sauce, canned	1 lg	39	24
Sardines, Pacific w/tomato sauce, canned	1 lg	39	24
Scallops, bay & sea; steamed	1 med	27	13
Sea Legs	3.5 oz	101	12
Shrimp; breaded, french fried	1 lg	18	11
Shrimp, canned	½ cup	64	82

FOOD	PORTION SIZE	CALORIES	CHOLESTEROL (Mg)
Shrimp jambalaya (Home recipe)	¾ cup	188	50
Sole, Baby, *Today's Catch* (Van de Kamp's)	4 oz	80	64
Trout, rainbow, fresh, whole	1 sm	222	63
Tuna casserole (Home recipe)	¾ cup	299	56
Tuna patty (Home recipe)	3½" cake	228	69
Tuna salad	½ cup	188	40
Tuna stuffed, green pepper (Home recipe)	1	261	59
Tuna, albacore, raw	3½ oz	177	60
Tuna, in water, canned (Generic)	½ cup	108	54
Tuna, in water, low sodium, canned (Generic)	½ cup	108	54
Tuna, in oil, canned (Generic)	½ cup	158	52
Tuna, in oil, canned (Generic)	7 oz can	333	110
Tuna, Chunk Light in Oil, canned (Star-Kist)	½ cup	225	50
Tuna, Chunk Light in Water, canned (Bumble Bee)	½ cup	117	58
Tuna, Chunk Light in Water, canned (Chicken Of The Sea)	½ cup	100	56
Tuna, Chunk White in Water, canned (Bumble Bee)	2 oz	70	30
Tuna, Solid White in Oil, canned (Bumble Bee)	2 oz	150	30
Tuna, Solid White in Water, canned (Bumble Bee)	2 oz	70	30
Tuna, Solid White in Water, canned (Bumble Bee)	½ cup	126	58
Tuna, Solid White in Water, canned (Star-Kist)	½ cup	110	58
Whiting Fillet, Today's Catch (Van de Kamp's)	4 oz	80	21

FOOD	PORTION SIZE	CALORIES	CHOLESTEROL (Mg)

FISH RESTAURANT MENU ITEMS
(see also individual fast food names)

All products below are from Fishery Products Inc. Many, but not all restaurants serve these or similar items. The items below have been included for comparative purposes only. Use them as a guide to judge the cholesterol in similar products.

FOOD	PORTION SIZE	CALORIES	CHOLESTEROL (Mg)
New England Style, Flounder, stuffed, Continental	7.5 oz	270	65
New England Style Scrod Cod	3.25 oz	163	43
New England Style Scrod Loins	2.5 oz	80	15
Prime Sea Strips, Crisp 'n Crunchy	4 oz	137	33
Prime Sea Strips, Home Style Batter	4.3 oz	172	52
Prime Sea Strips, Oven Style	4 oz	206	46
Prime Sea Strips, Southern Fried	4.3 oz	160	28
Sea Nuggets Country Oven Style Formed	3.5 oz	190	20
Sea Nuggets, Home Style Batter Natural Shaped	4.4 oz	180	45
Sea Nuggets, Oven Style Natural Fillet	4 oz	183	40
Sea Nuggets, Oven Style Natural Shaped	4.4 oz	220	40
Sea Nuggets, Southern Fried Natural Fillet	4.1 oz	152	27
Sea Nuggets, Southern Fried Natural Shaped	4.4 oz	140	40
Sea Nuggets, Specially Seasoned Formed	4 oz	240	26
Sea Nuggets, Specially Seasoned Natural Fillet	4.1 oz	211	27

FOOD	PORTION SIZE	CALORIES	CHOLESTEROL (Mg)
Sea Nuggets, Crisp 'n Crunchy Formed	4 oz	126	32
Sea Nuggets, Crisp'n Crunchy Natural Fillet	3.75 oz	129	30
Sea Nuggets, Sweet 'n Flaky Formed	4 oz	137	53
Sea Nuggets, Sweet 'n Flaky Natural Fillet	3.75 oz	129	25
Seafood Elites Scrod w/ Broccoli & Mozzarella	5 oz	140	66
Seafood Elites Scrod w/Lemon & Wild Rice	5 oz	150	49
Seafood Elites Scrod w/Spinach & Cheddar	5 oz	140	63
Seafood Elites Sole w/Broccoli & Mozzarella	5 oz	150	53
Seafood Elites Sole w/Lemon & Wild Rice	5 oz	150	47
Seafood Elites Sole w/Spinach & Cheddar	5 oz	130	58

FLOUR

Gold Medal Wondra	1 cup	400	none
Pillsbury's Best All Purpose Enriched	1 cup	400	none
Pillsbury's Best Whole Wheat, Graham	1 cup	400	none
Swans Down Cake Flour	¼ cup	100	none

FOOD	PORTION SIZE	CALORIES	CHOLESTEROL (Mg)

FRANKFURTER
(*see also* HAM, LUNCHEON MEATS/COLD CUTS, MEAT SUBSTITUTES, TURKEY)

FOOD	PORTION SIZE	CALORIES	CHOLESTEROL (Mg)
Beef & pork, frankfurter (Generic)	1	144	22
Beef Frank (Oscar Mayer)	1	144	27
Beef, frankfurter (Generic)	1	145	22
Beef, Hot dogs (Armour)	1	150	20
Beef, Our Old Fashioned Franks (Hillshire Farm)	3½ oz	311	24
Cheese Hot Dogs (Oscar Mayer)	1	145	30
Chicken frankfurter (Generic)	1	116	45
Chicken Franks (Tyson)	1	122	29
Chicken Franks (Weaver)	1	122	43
Nachos Style Cheese, Hot Dogs (Oscar Mayer)	1	138	30
Turkey Cheese Franks (Louis Rich)	1	108	39
Turkey frankfurter (Generic)	1	102	48
Turkey Franks (Empire)	1	120	65
Turkey Franks (Louis Rich)	1	103	40
Wieners (Oscar Mayer)	1	144	27
Weiners, Little (Oscar Mayer)	1 (9g)	28	5
Weiners w/Cheese (Oscar Mayer)	1	145	31

FRENCH FRIES
(*see* POTATOES)

FOOD	PORTION SIZE	CALORIES	CHOLESTEROL (Mg)

FRENCH TOAST
(*see also* CREPES, PANCAKES/HOT CAKES, WAFFLES)

FOOD	PORTION SIZE	CALORIES	CHOLESTEROL (Mg)
French Toast (Home recipe)	1 slice	155	122

FROG LEG

FOOD	PORTION SIZE	CALORIES	CHOLESTEROL (Mg)
Frog Leg; w/seasoned flour, fried (Home recipe)	1 med	70	12

FROZEN DINNERS
(*see also* CHICKEN, FROZEN PREPARED)

FOOD	PORTION SIZE	CALORIES	CHOLESTEROL (Mg)
Armour Chicken Fricassee Dinner Classic	11¾ oz	330	70
Armour Chicken Breast Marsala Dinner Classic Lite	11 oz	270	85
Armour Seafood Newburg Dinner Classic	10½ oz	270	90
Banquet International Favorites Veal Parmigiana Buffet Supper	6½ oz	277	85
Budget Gourmet Cheese Manicotti w/Meat Sauce	1 pkg	450	50
Budget Gourmet Chicken & Egg Noodles w/Broccoli	1 pkg	450	130
Budget Gourmet Chicken au Gratin	1 pkg	260	70
Budget Gourmet Chicken w/ Fettucini	1 pkg	400	100
Budget Gourmet Fettucini & Meat Sauce	1 pkg	290	25

FOOD	PORTION SIZE	CALORIES	CHOLESTEROL (Mg)
Budget Gourmet French Recipe Chicken	1 pkg	270	60
Budget Gourmet Italian Sausage Lasagna	1 pkg	420	80
Budget Gourmet Italian Style Meatballs & Noodles	1 pkg	310	55
Budget Gourmet Lasagna w/ Meat Sauce	1 pkg	290	25
Budget Gourmet Linguini w/Bay Shrimp & Clams Marinara	1 pkg	330	75
Budget Gourmet Linguini w/ Scallops & Clams	1 pkg	280	60
Budget Gourmet Mandarin Chicken	1 pkg	290	25
Budget Gourmet Oriental Beef	1 pkg	290	25
Budget Gourmet Pasta Shells & Beef	1 pkg	340	35
Budget Gourmet Pepper Steak w/Rice	1 pkg	300	25
Budget Gourmet Seafood Newburg	1 pkg	350	70
Budget Gourmet Sirloin of Beef in Herb Sauce	1 pkg	290	25
Budget Gourmet Sirloin Tips w/ Country Style Vegetables	1 pkg	310	40
Budget Gourmet Swedish Meatballs	1 pkg	600	140
Budget Gourmet Sweet & Sour Chicken w/Rice	1 pkg	350	40
Budget Gourmet Three Cheese Lasagna	1 pkg	400	65
Budget Gourmet Turkey a la King w/Rice	1 pkg	390	75

FOOD	PORTION SIZE	CALORIES	CHOLESTEROL (Mg)
El Charrito 2 Grande Beef Enchilada Dinner	16.5 oz	800	45
El Charrito 3 Beef Enchiladas	11 oz	560	55
El Charrito 3 Cheese Enchiladas	11 oz	470	30
El Charrito 3 Chicken Enchiladas	11 oz	440	60
El Charrito 4 Grande Beef Enchiladas	16.5	890	65
El Charrito 6 Beef & Cheese Enchiladas	16.25 oz	880	70
El Charrito 6 Beef Enchiladas	16.25 oz	880	75
El Charrito 6 Cheese Enchiladas	16.25 oz	780	45
El Charrito Beef Enchilada Dinner	13.75 oz	620	45
El Charrito Cheese Enchilada Dinner	13.75 oz	570	30
El Charrito Chicken Enchilada Dinner	13.75 oz	510	50
El Charrito Grande B&B Burrito	6 oz	430	25
El Charrito Grande Beef Enchilada Dinner	21 oz	950	70
El Charrito Grande Green Chile B&B Burrito	6 oz	410	20
El Charrito Grande Jalapeno Burrito	6 oz	410	25
El Charrito Grande Mexican Style Dinner	20 oz	850	65
El Charrito Grande Red Chile B&B Burrito	6 oz	410	25
El Charrito Grande Sattilo Dinner	20.75 oz	820	45
El Charrito Green Chile B&B Burrito	5 oz	370	20
El Charrito Mexican Style Dinner	14.25 oz	690	45

FOOD	PORTION SIZE	CALORIES	CHOLESTEROL (Mg)
El Charrito Queso Dinner	13.25 oz	490	15
El Charrito Red Chile B&B Burrito	5 oz	380	20
El Charrito Red Hot B&B Burrito	5 oz	540	20
El Charrito Red Hot Beef Burrito	5 oz	340	20
El Charrito Sattilo Dinner	13.75 oz	570	30
Morton Beef Patty Boil-In-Bag Entree	5 oz	200	35
Morton Beef Pot Pie	8 oz	320	40
Morton Creamed Chipped Beef Boil-In-Bag Entree	5 oz	160	17
Morton Fried Chicken Dinner	11 oz	460	84
Morton Sloppy Joe Boil-In-Bag Entree	5 oz	210	33
Morton Turkey Dinner	11 oz	340	66
Morton Turkey Pot Pie	8 oz	340	45
Morton Veal Parmigiana Dinner	11 oz	250	36
Stouffer's Lean Cuisine Beef & Pork Cannelloni w/Mornay Sauce	9⅝ oz	270	50
Stouffer's Lean Cuisine Breast of Chicken Marsala w/ Vegetables	8⅛ oz	190	60
Stouffer's Lean Cuisine Cheese Cannelloni w/Tomato Sauce	9⅛ oz	270	35
Stouffer's Lean Cuisine Chicken Cacciatore w/Vermicelli	10⅞ oz	280	55
Stouffer's Lean Cuisine Chicken a l'Orange w/Almond Rice	8 oz	270	55
Stouffer's Lean Cuisine Chicken & Vegetable w/Vermicelli	12¾ oz	270	50
Stouffer's Lean Cuisine Chicken Chow Mein w/Rice	11¼ oz	250	35

FOOD	PORTION SIZE	CALORIES	CHOLESTEROL (Mg)
Stouffer's Lean Cuisine Filet of Fish Divan	12⅜ oz	270	95
Stouffer's Lean Cuisine Filet of Fish Florentine	9 oz	240	90
Stouffer's Lean Cuisine Filet of Fish Jardiniere w/Souffleed Potatoes	11¼ oz	280	110
Stouffer's Lean Cuisine Glazed Chicken w/Vegetable Rice	8½ oz	270	65
Stouffer's Lean Cuisine Herbed Lamb w/Rice	10⅜ oz	280	70
Stouffer's Lean Cuisine Linguini w/Clam Sauce	9⅝ oz	260	35
Stouffer's Lean Cuisine Meatball Stew	10 oz	250	80
Stouffer's Lean Cuisine Oriental Beef w/Vegetables & Rice	8⅝ oz	270	45
Stouffer's Lean Cuisine Oriental Scallops & Vegetables w/Rice	11 oz	220	20
Stouffer's Lean Cuisine Salisbury Steak w/Italian Style Sauce & Vegetables	9½ oz	270	110
Stouffer's Lean Cuisine Shrimp & Chicken Cantonese w/Noodles	10⅛ oz	270	130
Stouffer's Lean Cuisine Spaghetti w/Beef & Mushroom Sauce	11½ oz	280	30
Stouffer's Lean Cuisine Stuffed Cabbage w/Meat in Tomato Sauce	10¾ oz	220	45
Stouffer's Lean Cuisine Tuna Lasagna w/Spinach Noodles & Vegetables	9¾ oz	280	25

FOOD	PORTION SIZE	CALORIES	CHOLESTEROL (Mg)
Stouffer's Lean Cuisine Turkey Dijon	9½ oz	280	70
Stouffer's Lean Cuisine Veal Lasagna	10¼ oz	280	90
Stouffer's Lean Cuisine Veal Primavera	9⅛ oz	250	90
Stouffer's Lean Cuisine Zucchini Lasagna	11 oz	260	25
Swanson Fried Chicken Dinner	1 dinner	583	184
Tyson Chick'n Quick, Thick and Crispy Dinner Patties	7 oz	560	106
Tyson Heat'n Serve Oven Ready Fully Cooked Chicken	7 oz	540	148

FRUIT
(*see also* FRUIT DRINKS, FRUIT SNACKS, JUICE)

FOOD	PORTION SIZE	CALORIES	CHOLESTEROL (Mg)
Apple	1 med	81	none
Applesauce (Mott's)	½ cup	115	none
Applesauce, unsweetened, *Musselman* (Knouse Foods)	½ cup	50	none
Apricots, dried	10 halves	83	none
Apricots, raw	3 med	51	none
Banana	1 med	105	none
Blackberries	½ cup	37	none
Blueberries	1 cup	82	none
Cantaloupe, diced	1 cup	57	none
Cherries	10	49	none
Cranberries, raw	1 cup	46	none
Cranberry sauce	½ cup	200	none
Dates	10	228	none
Figs	1 med	37	none
Fruit Cocktail (Del Monte)	½ cup	80	none

FOOD	PORTION SIZE	CALORIES	CHOLESTEROL (Mg)
Fruit Cocktail (Libby's)	½ cup	85	none
Grapefruit	½ med	37	none
Grapes	1 cup	58	none
Honeydew	¼ sm	33	none
Kiwi fruit	1 med	46	none
Lemon	1 med	17	none
Lime	1 med	20	none
Lychees	10 med	66	none
Mango	1 med	135	none
Orange navel	1 med	65	none
Orange, Mandarin, In Light Syrup (Dole)	½ cup	76	none
Peach	1 med	37	none
Peach Halves, Yellow Cling (Del Monte)	½ cup	50	none
Peaches, Yellow Cling, *Lite, in Fruit Juice* (Libby's)	½ cup	50	none
Pear	1 med	98	none
Pear Halves, Bartlett (Del Monte)	½ cup	80	none
Persimmon	1 med	32	none
Pineapple	1 cup	77	none
Pineapple, Sliced, In Juice (Dole)	½ cup	70	none
Pineapple, Sliced, In Syrup (Dole)	½ cup	95	none
Plum	1 med	36	none
Prunes (Sunsweet)	5	120	none
Raisins, Seedless (Sun-Maid)	⅓ cup	192	none
Raspberries	1 cup	61	none
Strawberries, In Syrup, frzn (Birds Eye)	½ cup	100	none
Tangerine	1 med	37	none
Watermelon	1 cup	50	none

FOOD	PORTION SIZE	CALORIES	CHOLESTEROL (Mg)
FRUIT DRINKS (*see also* JUICE)			
Cranberry apple juice drink (Generic)	8 oz	160	none
Cranberry apricot juice drink (Generic)	8 oz	160	none
Cranberry grape juice drink (Generic)	8 oz	136	none
Cranberry juice cocktail (Generic)	8 oz	144	none
Fruit Punch, *Capri Sun* (Consolidated Food, Inc)	6¾ oz	102	none
Fruit punch, canned (Generic)	8 oz	112	none
Fruit punch, frzn; as prep w/ water	8 oz	112	none
Fruit punch, powder (Generic)	2 Tbsp	97	none
Fruit Punch, *Hi-C*	12 oz	154	none
Fruit Punch, Grape, *Hi-C*	12 oz	154	none
Fruit Punch, *Hawaiian Punch* (R.J. Reynolds)	6 oz	84	none
Fruit Punch, Lemon, *Hi-C*	12 oz	142	none
Fruit Punch, Orange, *Hi-C*	12 oz	152	none
Fruit punch, thirst quencher drink, bottled (Generic)	8 oz	56	none
Lemonade; as prep w/water (Generic)	8 oz	104	none
Lemonade, frzn concentrate; as prep w/water (Generic)	8 oz	104	none
Lemonade, powder (Generic)	2 Tbsp	113	none
Limeade, frzn concentrate; as prep w/water (Generic)	8 oz	104	none
Orange & apricot juice drink, canned (Generic)	8 oz	128	none
Orange drink, canned (Generic)	8 oz	128	none

FOOD	PORTION SIZE	CALORIES	CHOLESTEROL (Mg)
Orange flavor drink, breakfast type, frzn concentrate (Generic)	8 oz	120	none
Orange flavor drink, breakfast type, powder (Generic)	3 tsp	93	none
Pineapple & grapefruit juice drink, canned (Generic)	8 oz	120	none
Pineapple & orange juice drink, canned (Generic)	8 oz	128	none

FRUIT SNACKS

FOOD	PORTION SIZE	CALORIES	CHOLESTEROL (Mg)
Fun Fruits, all flavors (Sun Kist)	1 pkg	100	none
Fun Fruits, animals or numbers (Sun Kist)	1 pkg	100	none
Fruit Roll-Ups, all flavors (General Mills)	1 roll	50	none
Fruit Wrinkles, all flavors (General Mills)	1 pkg	100	none

GIBLETS

FOOD	PORTION SIZE	CALORIES	CHOLESTEROL (Mg)
Chicken; floured, fried	1 chicken	208	335
Chicken; simmered	¼ cup	55	143
Chicken; stewed, chopped	½ cup	114	285
Turkey; simmered	¼ cup	61	152

GIZZARD

FOOD	PORTION SIZE	CALORIES	CHOLESTEROL (Mg)
Chicken; cooked	¼ cup	56	70
Chicken; stewed	1	31	39
Turkey; cooked	¼ cup	59	84
Turkey; stewed, chopped	½ cup	118	168

FOOD	PORTION SIZE	CALORIES	CHOLESTEROL (Mg)

GOOSE

Liver pate, smoked, canned	1 Tbsp	60	19
W/skin; cooked	¼ lb	600	43
W/o skin; cooked	¼ lb	356	34

GRANOLA BAR

Oats 'N Honey *Nature Valley* (General Mills)	1 bar (0.8 oz)	110	none
W/Roasted Almonds, *Nature Valley* (General Mills)	1 bar (0.8 oz)	120	none

GRAVY (*see also* DIPS; SALAD DRESSINGS; SOUPS, DRY)

Canned, au jus (Generic)	¼ cup	10	tr
Canned, beef (Generic)	¼ cup	31	2
Canned, chicken (Generic)	¼ cup	47	1
Canned, mushroom (Generic)	¼ cup	30	none
Canned, turkey (Generic)	¼ cup	30	1
Dry, au jus (Generic)	⅘ oz pkg	79	4
Dry, au jus; as prep w/water (Generic)	¼ cup	5	tr
Dry, brown (Generic)	⅞ oz pkg	85	2
Dry, brown; as prep w/water (Generic)	¼ cup	2	tr
Dry, chicken (Generic)	⅘ oz pkg	83	2
Dry, chicken; as prep w/water (Generic)	¼ cup	21	1
Dry, mushroom (Generic)	¾ oz pkg	70	1
Dry, mushroom; as prep w/ water (Generic)	¼ cup	17	tr
Dry, onion (Generic)	⅚ oz pkg	77	none

FOOD	PORTION SIZE	CALORIES	CHOLESTEROL (Mg)
Dry, onion; as prep w/water (Generic)	¼ cup	20	none
Dry, pork (Generic)	¾ oz pkg	76	2
Dry, pork; as prep w/water (Generic)	¼ cup	19	1
Dry, turkey (Generic)	⅞ oz pkg	87	2
Dry, turkey; as prep w/water (Generic)	¼ cup	22	1

HAM (*see also* FRANKFURTER, LUNCHEON MEATS/COLD CUTS, MEAT SUBSTITUTES, TURKEY)

FOOD	PORTION SIZE	CALORIES	CHOLESTEROL (Mg)
Canned, chopped (Generic)	1 oz	68	14
Canned, *Golden Star* (Armour)	2 oz	60	33
Chopped (Generic)	1 oz	65	15
Ham (Land O' Frost)	2 oz	100	33
Honey Ham w/Natural Juices (Oscar Mayer)	1 slice	27	11
Italian Style Cooked w/Natural Juices (Oscar Mayer)	1 slice	24	9
Jubilee (Oscar Mayer)	1 oz	31	13
Jubilee, Boneless (Oscar Mayer)	1 oz	47	15
Jubilee, Sliced (Oscar Mayer)	1 oz	29	13
Jubilee Steaks (Oscar Mayer)	2 oz	59	27
Minced (Generic)	1 oz	75	20
Patty; grilled	2 oz	203	43
Sliced, extra lean (Generic)	1 slice	74	27
Sliced, regular (Generic)	1 slice	52	16
Smoked (Oscar Mayer)	3 oz	102	35
Smoked center slice, w/o bone, fully trimmed (Generic)	3 oz	159	75
Smoked, center slice, w/o bone, not trimmed (Generic)	3 oz	246	76

FOOD	PORTION SIZE	CALORIES	CHOLESTEROL (Mg)
Smoked, chopped, fully trimmed (Generic)	½ cup	131	62
Smoked, ground, not trimmed (Generic)	½ cup	159	49
Smoked w/natural juices (Generic)	1 slice	23	10
Smoked, w/o bone, cubed, fully trimmed (Generic)	½ cup	131	62
Smoked, w/o bone, cubed, not trimmed (Generic)	½ cup	202	62

HAMBURGER HELPER (*see* BEEF)

HARDEE'S

FOOD	PORTION SIZE	CALORIES	CHOLESTEROL (Mg)
Apple Turnover	1	282	5
Bacon Cheeseburger	1	556	60
Biscuit, Bacon & Egg	1	405	305
Biscuit, *Cinnamon 'N' Raisin*	1	276	tr
Biscuit, Country Ham	1	328	12
Biscuit, Egg	1	334	160
Biscuit, Gravy	1	144	21
Biscuit, Ham & Egg	1	458	293
Biscuit, Sausage	1	413	29
Biscuit, Sausage & Egg	1	521	293
Biscuit, Steak	1	419	34
Biscuit, Steak & Egg	1	527	298
Biscuit, Sugar Cured Ham	1	299	17
Big Cookie	1	278	9
Big Country Breakfast Platter, Bacon	1	716	350
Big Country Breakfast Platter, Ham	1	665	369

FOOD	PORTION SIZE	CALORIES	CHOLESTEROL (Mg)
Big Country Breakfast Platter, Sausage	1	940	442
Big Deluxe	1	503	50
Big Roast Beef	1	440	86
Canadian Sunrise	1	482	255
Cheeseburger	1	309	28
Chef Salad	1	277	179
Chicken Fillet	1	510	57
Fisherman's Fillet	1	469	80
French Fries, lg	1	381	6
French Fries, reg	1	239	4
Hamburger	1	276	22
Hash Rounds	1	200	10
Hot Dog	1	346	42
Hot Ham 'N' Cheese	1	376	59
Milkshake	1	391	42
Mushroom 'N' Swiss	1	512	86
¼ Pound Cheeseburger	1	511	77
Roast Beef Sandwich	1	312	68
Turkey Club	1	426	45

HEART

Beef; braised, chopped	½ cup	136	199
Beef; cooked	3 oz	148	164
Chicken; cooked	1	6	7
Chicken; cooked	¼ cup	67	88
Turkey; cooked	¼ cup	64	82
Turkey; stewed, chopped	½ cup	128	164

HONEY

	1 Tbsp	61	none

FOOD	PORTION SIZE	CALORIES	CHOLESTEROL (Mg)

HOT CAKES
(*see* PANCAKES/HOT CAKES)

HOT DOGS
(*see* FRANKFURTER)

ICE CREAM & FROZEN DESSERTS
(*see also* DAIRY QUEEN; PUDDING POP; YOGURT, FROZEN)

FOOD	PORTION SIZE	CALORIES	CHOLESTEROL (Mg)
Banana, *Fruit 'N Juice Bars* (Dole)	1 bar	80	none
Blueberry, *Fruit and Cream Bars* (Dole)	1 bar	90	5
Cappuccino, *Love Drops, Tofutti*	4 oz	230	none
Chocolate, *Cuties, Tofutti*	1	140	none
Chocolate, *Love Drops, Tofutti*	4 oz	230	none
Chocolate, *Soft Serve, Tofutti Hi-Lite*	4 oz	100	none
Chocolate, *Supreme, Tofutti*	4 oz	210	none
Fruit, Sherbert (Land O Lakes)	4 oz	130	5
Mandarin Orange, Sorbet (Dole)	4 oz	110	none
Orange, sherbet (Generic)	1 cup	270	14
Orange w/ Mandarin, *Fruit 'N Juice Bars* (Dole)	1 bar	70	none
Peach, *Fruit and Cream Bars* (Dole)	1 bar	90	5
Peach, Sorbet (Dole)	4 oz	120	none
Pina Colada, *Fruit 'N Juice Bars* (Dole)	1 bar	90	none

FOOD	PORTION SIZE	CALORIES	CHOLESTEROL (Mg)
Pineapple, *Fruit 'N Juice Bars* (Dole)	1 bar	70	none
Pineapple, Sorbet (Dole)	4 oz	120	none
Raspberry, *Fruit 'N Juice Bars* (Dole)	1 bar	70	none
Raspberry, Sorbet (Dole)	4 oz	110	none
Strawberry, *Fruit and Cream Bars* (Dole)	1 bar	90	5
Strawberry, *Fruit 'N Juice Bars* (Dole)	1 bar	70	none
Strawberry, Sorbet (Dole)	4 oz	110	none
Vanilla, Almond Bark, *Tofutti*	4 oz	230	none
Vanilla Blueberry Swirl (Carnation)	1.7 oz	70	9
Vanilla, *Cuties, Tofutti*	1	130	none
Vanilla, French, soft serve (Generic)	1 cup	377	153
Vanilla, Frzn Dietary Dairy Dessert (Sugar Lo)	2.6 oz	90	5
Vanilla, Ice Cream (Land O Lakes)	4 oz	140	30
Vanilla ice cream, regular, 10% fat (Generic)	1 cup	269	59
Vanilla ice cream, rich, 16% fat (Generic)	1 cup	349	88
Vanilla ice milk (Generic)	1 cup	184	18
Vanilla, Ice Milk (Land O Lakes)	4 oz	90	10
Vanilla Ice Milk, *Light N' Lively* (Sealtest)	4 oz	100	5
Vanilla ice milk, soft serve (Generic)	1 cup	223	13
Vanilla, *Love Drops, Tofutti*	4 oz	220	none
Vanilla, *Soft Serve, Tofutti*	4 oz	158	none

FOOD	PORTION SIZE	CALORIES	CHOLESTEROL (Mg)
Vanilla, *Soft Serve, Tofutti Hi-Lite*	4 oz	90	none
Vanilla, *Tasti-D-Lite*	6 oz	60	15
Vanilla, *Tofutti*	4 oz	200	none
Wildberry, *Tofutti*	4 oz	210	none

ICING

Chocolate (Home recipe)	1 cup	1123	75
Coconut fluff (Home recipe)	1 cup	533	77
White, boiled (Home recipe)	1 cup	247	none
White, uncooked (Home recipe)	1 cup	813	60

INSTANT BREAKFAST
(*see* NUTRITIONAL SUPPLEMENTS)

JACK IN THE BOX

Apple Turnover	1	410	15
Bacon Cheeseburger Supreme	1	724	70
Breakfast Jack	1	307	203
Canadian Crescent	1	472	226
Cheese Nachos	1	571	37
Cheeseburger	1	323	42
Chicken Strips Dinner	1	689	100
Chicken Supreme	1	601	60
Chocolate Shake	1	330	25
Club Pita	1	284	43
Cooked Bacon	2 slices	70	10

FOOD	PORTION SIZE	CALORIES	CHOLESTEROL (Mg)
French Fries, reg	1 portion	221	8
Ham & Swiss Burger	1	638	117
Hamburger	1	276	29
Hash Brown Potatoes	1 portion	68	none
Jumbo Jack	1	485	64
Jumbo Jack w/cheese	1	630	110
Moby Jack	1	444	47
Mushroom Burger	1	477	87
Onion Rings	1 portion	382	27
Pancakes Breakfast	1	626	85
Pasta Seafood Salad	1	394	48
Regular Taco	1	191	21
Sausage Crescent	1	584	187
Scrambled Eggs Breakfast	1	719	260
Shrimp Dinner	1	731	157
Sirloin Steak Dinner	1	699	75
Strawberry Shake	1	320	25
Super Taco	1	288	37
Supreme Crescent	1	547	178
Supreme Nachos	1	718	65
Swiss & Bacon Burger	1	643	99
Taco Salad	1	377	102
Vanilla Shake	1	320	25

JAM/JELLY

FOOD	PORTION SIZE	CALORIES	CHOLESTEROL (Mg)
All Fruit Spreadable Fruits (Polaner)	1 tsp	14	none
All varieties (Generic)	1 Tbsp	50	none
Fruit Only Conserve; all flavors (Sorrel Ridge)	1 tsp	14	none
Imitation Grape Jelly (Smucker's)	2 Tbsp	4	none

FOOD	PORTION SIZE	CALORIES	CHOLESTEROL (Mg)

JUICE
(*see also* FRUIT DRINKS)

FOOD	PORTION SIZE	CALORIES	CHOLESTEROL (Mg)
Apple	8 oz	116	none
Grapefruit	8 oz	96	none
Orange	8 oz	111	none
Pineapple	8 oz	139	none
Tomato	8 oz	41	none

KETCHUP
(*see* CATSUP)

KENTUCKY FRIED CHICKEN

CHICKEN DISHES

FOOD	PORTION SIZE	CALORIES	CHOLESTEROL (Mg)
Extra Crispy, Center Breast	1	353	93
Extra Crispy, Drumstick	1	173	65
Extra Crispy, Side Breast	1	354	66
Extra Crispy, Thigh	1	371	121
Extra Crispy, Wing	1	218	63
Original, Center Breast	1	257	93
Original, Drumstick	1	147	81
Original, Side Breast	1	276	96
Original, Thigh	1	278	122
Original, Wing	1	181	67
Kentucky Nuggets	1	46	12
Kentucky Nugget Sauce, Barbecue	1 oz	35	1
Kentucky Nugget Sauce, Honey	1 oz	49	1
Kentucky Nugget Sauce, Mustard	1 oz	36	1
Kentucky Nugget Sauce, Sweet and Sour	1 oz	58	1

FOOD	PORTION SIZE	CALORIES	CHOLESTEROL (Mg)

SIDE DISHES

Baked Beans	1 portion	105	1
Buttermilk Biscuit	1	269	1
Chicken Gravy	1	59	2
Cole Slaw	1	103	4
Corn On The Cob		176	1
Kentucky Fries	1	268	2
Mashed Potatoes	1	59	1
Mashed Potatoes w/Gravy	1	62	1
Potato Salad	1	141	11

KIDNEY

Beef; braised	1 slice	252	375
Beef; simmered	3 oz	122	329
Pork; cooked	3 oz	128	408

LAMB

Curry (Home recipe)	¾ cup	345	89
Ground, not trimmed; cooked	½ cup	153	54
Leg, w/o bone, fully trimmed; roasted	2 slices	158	85
Leg, w/o bone, not trimmed; roasted	2 slices	237	83
Loin chop, w/bone, fully trimmed; broiled	1 med (4 oz)	92	49
Loin chop, w/bone, not trimmed; broiled	1 med (4 oz)	255	70
Patty; cooked	3 oz	229	80
Potato casserole (Home recipe)	¾ cup	277	58
Rib chop, w/bone, fully trimmed; broiled	1 med (4 oz)	91	43

FOOD	PORTION SIZE	CALORIES	CHOLESTEROL (Mg)
Rib chop, w/bone, not trimmed; broiled	1 med (4 oz)	273	66
Shoulder shank, not trimmed; cooked	½ shank	306	89
Shoulder, w/o bone, fully trimmed; roasted	3 slices 2½″ sq × ¼″ each	174	85
Shoulder, w/o bone, not trimmed; roasted	3 slices 2½″ sq × ¼″ each	287	83

LARD
(*see* FATS)

LIQUOR/LIQUEURS
(*see also* BEER, WINE)

FOOD	PORTION SIZE	CALORIES	CHOLESTEROL (Mg)
Anisette	⅔ oz	74	none
Apricot brandy	⅔ oz	64	none
Benedictine	⅔ oz	69	none
Brandy	1 oz	73	none
Cider, fermented	6 oz	73	none
Cognac	⅔ oz	75	none
Creme de menthe	⅔ oz	67	none
Curacao	⅔ oz	54	none
Daiquiri	2½ oz	87	none
Gin, 80 proof	1½ oz	97	none
Manhattan	2½ oz	116	none
Martini	2½ oz	99	none
Mint julep	10 oz	210	none
Old Fashioned	2½ oz	127	none
Rum, 80 proof	1½ oz	105	none
Scotch	1½ oz	107	none

FOOD	PORTION SIZE	CALORIES	CHOLESTEROL (Mg)
Sloe Gin Fizz	2½ oz	132	none
Tom Collins	10 oz	180	none
Vodka, 80 proof	1½ oz	97	none
Whiskey, 86 proof	1½ oz	97	none

LIVER

FOOD	PORTION SIZE	CALORIES	CHOLESTEROL (Mg)
Beef; cooked	3 oz	150	372
Beef; fried	3 oz	195	372
Calve's; cooked	3 oz	166	372
Chicken; stewed	1	39	158
Chicken; stewed, chopped	½ cup	110	442
Duck	1 raw (44g)	60	227
Goose pate, smoked, canned	1 Tbsp	60	19
Mushroom & liver casserole (Home recipe)	¾ cup	208	157
Turkey; stewed, chopped	½ cup	118	438

LONG JOHN SILVER'S

FOOD	PORTION SIZE	CALORIES	CHOLESTEROL (Mg)
Batter Fried Fish	1	202	31
Batter Fried Shrimp	1	47	17
Batter Fried Shrimp Dinner	1	711	127
Clam Chowder	1	128	17
Clam Dinner	1	955	27
Cole Slaw	1	182	12
Fish & Chicken	1	935	56
Fish & More	1	978	88
Fish Sandwich Platter	1	835	75
Fryes	1	247	13
Hush Puppies	1	145	1

FOOD	PORTION SIZE	CALORIES	CHOLESTEROL (Mg)
Kitchen Breaded Fish	1	122	25
Ocean Chef Salad	1	229	64
Oyster Dinner	1	789	55
2 Piece Fish & *Fryes*	1	651	75
2 Piece Kitchen Breaded Fish Dinner	1	818	76
3 Piece Chicken Planks Dinner	1	885	25
3 Piece Fish & *Fryes*	1	853	106
3 Piece Fish Dinner	1	1180	119
3 Piece Kitchen Breaded Fish Dinner	1	940	101
4 Piece Chicken Planks Dinner	1	1037	25
6 Piece Chicken Nuggets Dinner	1	699	25
Scallop Dinner	1	747	37
Seafood Platter	1	976	95
Seafood Salad	1	426	113

LUNCHEON MEATS/COLD CUTS

(*see also* FRANKFURTER, HAM, MEAT SUBSTITUTES, SAUSAGE, TURKEY)

FOOD	PORTION SIZE	CALORIES	CHOLESTEROL (Mg)
Bar-B-Q Loaf (Oscar Mayer)	1 slice (28 g)	7	3
Barbecue loaf, pork & beef (Generic)	1 slice	40	9
Beef, Smoked (Buddig)	1 oz	42	16
Beerwurst, beef (Generic)	1 slice	75	13
Beerwurst, pork (Generic)	1 slice	55	13
Berliner, pork & beef (Generic)	1 slice	53	11
Blood sausage (Generic)	1 slice	95	30
Bologna (Generic)	1 slice	86	18
Bologna (Oscar Mayer)	1 slice (23 g)	74	13
Bologna, All Meat (Oscar Mayer)	1 slice	89	15

FOOD	PORTION SIZE	CALORIES	CHOLESTEROL (Mg)
Bologna, Beef (Armour)	2 slices (1 oz each)	180	30
Bologna, Beef (Oscar Mayer)	1 slice (23 g)	74	12
Bologna, beef & pork (Generic)	1 slice	73	13
Bologna, Beef, Lebanon (Oscar Mayer)	1 link (45 g)	50	16
Bologna, Garlic Beef (Oscar Mayer)	1 slice (23 g)	73	13
Bologna, ground (Generic)	2 Tbsp	86	18
Bologna, pork (Generic)	1 slice	57	14
Bologna, Pure Beef (Oscar Mayer)	1 slice	89	16
Bologna, turkey (Generic)	1 slice	57	28
Bologna With Cheese (Oscar Mayer)	1 slice (23 g)	74	14
Bratwurst, pork (Generic)	1 oz	85	17
Braunschweiger, German Brand (Oscar Mayer)	1 slice (1 oz)	94	46
Braunschweiger, Liver Sausage (Oscar Mayer)	1 slice (28 g)	95	50
Braunschweiger, smoked liver sausage (Generic)	1 slice	89	17
Chicken roll, light meat (Generic)	6 oz	271	85
Chicken, Smoked (Buddig)	1 oz	50	12
Corn beef loaf, jellied (Generic)	1 oz	46	12
Corned Beef (Buddig)	1 oz	42	16
Corned Beef (Oscar Mayer)	1 slice (17 g)	16	5
Ham & cheese loaf (Generic)	1 slice	73	16
Ham & Cheese Loaf (Oscar Mayer)	1 slice (1 oz)	77	16

FOOD	PORTION SIZE	CALORIES	CHOLESTEROL (Mg)
Ham & cheese spread (Generic)	1 Tbsp	37	9
Ham salad spread (Home recipe)	1 oz	62	11
Ham salad spread (Home recipe)	1 Tbsp	32	6
Ham, boiled (Generic)	6 × 4″ slice	66	25
Ham, chipped (Generic)	1 slice	68	20
Ham, Chopped (Oscar Mayer)	1 slice	61	14
Ham, Cooked (Oscar Mayer)	1 oz	34	17
Ham, Cracked Black Pepper (Oscar Mayer)	1 slice	24	11
Ham, Smoked (Buddig)	1 oz	49	20
Headcheese (Generic)	1 oz	60	23
Headcheese (Oscar Mayer)	1 slice (1 oz)	55	21
Honey Loaf (Oscar Mayer)	1 slice (1 oz)	35	12
Honey loaf, pork & beef (Generic)	1 slice	36	10
Italian Style Beef (Oscar Mayer)	1 slice (17 g)	18	6
Knockwurst, pork (Generic)	4″ link	189	42
Liver Cheese Pork Fat Wrap (Oscar Mayer)	1 slice (38 g)	116	75
Liverwurst, fresh (Generic)	2 Tbsp	86	29
Liverwurst, fresh, sliced (Generic)	1 oz	87	30
Luncheon Loaf, Turkey (Louis Rich)	1 oz	43	14
Luncheon Meat (Oscar Mayer)	1 slice (1 oz)	99	16
Luncheon meat, pork & ham (Generic)	1 Tbsp	83	25

FOOD	PORTION SIZE	CALORIES	CHOLESTEROL (Mg)
Luxury Loaf (Oscar Mayer)	1 slice (1 oz)	38	13
Luxury loaf, pork (Generic)	1 oz	40	10
Old Fashioned Loaf (Oscar Mayer)	1 slice (1 oz)	64	14
Olive Loaf (Oscar Mayer)	1 slice (1 oz)	63	10
Olive loaf, pork (Generic)	1 oz	67	11
Pastrami (Oscar Mayer)	1 slice (17 g)	17	5
Pastrami, Smoked (Buddig)	1 oz	42	16
Peppered Loaf (Oscar Mayer)	1 slice (1 oz)	43	13
Peppered loaf, pork & beef (Generic)	1 oz	42	13
Phrasky beef	2 thin slices	87	17
Pickle & pimento loaf (Generic)	1 oz	74	10
Pickle & Pimento Loaf (Oscar Mayer)	1 slice (1 oz)	64	10
Picnic Loaf (Oscar Mayer)	1 slice (1 oz)	62	12
Picnic loaf, pork (Generic)	1 oz	66	11
Salami beef (Generic)	4½" diam slice (1 oz)	87	17
Salami, Cotto (Oscar Mayer)	1 slice (23 g)	54	15
Salami, Cotto, Beef (Oscar Mayer)	1 slice (23 g)	45	15
Salami, Cotto, Turkey (Louis Rich)	1 oz	52	22
Salami, For Beer (Oscar Mayer)	1 slice (23 g)	55	15
Salami for Beer, Beef (Oscar Mayer)	1 slice (23 g)	67	21

FOOD	PORTION SIZE	CALORIES	CHOLESTEROL (Mg)
Salami, Genoa (Oscar Mayer)	1 slice (9 g)	35	8
Salami, Hard (Oscar Mayer)	1 slice (9 g)	34	7
Salami, hard, beef (Generic)	2 thin slices	126	17
Salami, Turkey (Generic)	3¼ × ⅛"	56	23
Sandwich Spread (Oscar Mayer)	1 Tbsp	34	5
Sandwich spread, poultry (Generic)	1 Tbsp	26	4
Spam. Pressed Meat (Hormel)	1 oz	88	25
Spiced meat, pork & ham (Generic)	4 × 3 × ⅛" slice	82	25
Summer Sausage, Beef, Thuringer Cervelat (Generic)	1 slice (23 g)	70	17
Summer Sausage, Beef, Thuringer Cervelat (Oscar Mayer)	1 slice (23 g)	73	17
Summer Sausage, Thuringer, Cervelat (Oscar Mayer)	1 slice (23 g)	73	17
Turkey Ham, Smoked (Buddig)	1 oz	40	19
Turkey roll, light & dark meat (Generic)	1 oz	24	16
Turkey roll, light meat (Generic)	1 oz	42	16
Turkey, Smoked (Buddig)	1 oz	47	6

MARGARINE
(*see also* BUTTER, FATS, MAYONNAISE, OILS)

FOOD	PORTION SIZE	CALORIES	CHOLESTEROL (Mg)
Diet Imitation (Mazola)	1 Tbsp	50	none
Diet, Light Spread, Corn oil (Parkay)	1 Tbsp	70	none
Diet, Light Spread, 50% Fat (Parkay)	1 Tbsp	60	none

FOOD	PORTION SIZE	CALORIES	CHOLESTEROL (Mg)
Diet Margarine (Fleischmann's)	1 Tbsp	50	none
Diet, Reduced Calorie (Parkay)	1 Tbsp	50	none
Diet, Reduced Calorie, Quarters (Weight Watchers)	1 Tbsp	60	none
Diet, Reduced Calorie, Tub (Weight Watchers)	1 Tbsp	50	none
Regular (Blue Bonnet)	1 Tbsp	102	none
Regular (Chiffon)	1 Tbsp	68	none
Regular (Fleischmann's)	1 Tbsp	102	none
Regular (Generic)	1 Tbsp	101	none
Regular, (Krona)	1 Tbsp	100	15
Regular (Parkay)	1 Tbsp	100	none
Regular (Promise)	1 Tbsp	93	none
Regular, Corn Oil, *Premium* (Land O Lakes)	1 Tbsp	100	none
Regular, Corn Oil (Mrs. Filbert's)	1 Tbsp	102	none
Regular, Corn Oil (Mazola)	1 Tbsp	101	none
Regular, Corn Oil (Parkay)	1 Tbsp	100	none
Regular Corn Oil, Soft (Mrs. Filbert's)	1 Tbsp	102	none
Regular, Corn Oil, Unsalted (Mazola)	1 Tbsp	100	none
Regular, Lightly Salted, *Country Morning Blend* (Land O Lakes)	1 Tbsp	100	10
Regular, Salted (Mother's)	1 Tbsp	100	none
Regular Soft (Promise)	1 Tbsp	102	none
Regular, Soy Oil (Land O Lakes)	1 Tbsp	100	none
Regular, Unsalted *Country Morning Blend* (Land O Lakes)	1 Tbsp	100	10
Regular, Unsalted (Mother's)	1 Tbsp	100	none

FOOD	PORTION SIZE	CALORIES	CHOLESTEROL (Mg)
Soft (Parkay)	1 Tbsp	100	none
Soft, Corn Oil (Parkay)	1 Tbsp	100	none
Soft, *Family Spread* (Mrs. Filbert's)	1 Tbsp	70	none
Soft, Lightly Salted *Country Morning Blend* (Land O Lakes)	1 Tbsp	90	10
Soft, *Miracle Brand* (Kraft)	1 Tbsp	60	none
Soft, Salted (Mother's)	1 Tbsp	100	none
Soft, Unsalted (Mother's)	1 Tbsp	100	none
Soft, Unsalted *Country Morning Blend* (Land O Lakes)	1 Tbsp	90	10
Squeeze (Parkay)	1 Tbsp	100	none
Whipped (Generic)	1 Tbsp	67	none
Whipped, Tub or Stick (Parkay)	1 Tbsp	60	none

MARSHMALLOW

MARSHMALLOW	1 med	25	none

MAYONNAISE
(*see also* BUTTER, FATS, MARGARINE, OILS)

FOOD	PORTION SIZE	CALORIES	CHOLESTEROL (Mg)
Regular (Mother's)	1 Tbsp	100	10
Regular, *Blue Plate* (William B. Reilly and Co)	1 Tbsp	100	10
Regular, *Miracle Whip Salad Dressing* (Kraft)	1 Tbsp	70	5
Regular, Real Mayonnaise (Kraft)	1 Tbsp	100	5
Regular, Real Mayonnaise, Best Foods (CPC International, Inc)	1 Tbsp	100	7

FOOD	PORTION SIZE	CALORIES	CHOLESTEROL (Mg)
Regular *Real Mayonnaise, Hellmann's* (CPC International, Inc)	1 Tbsp	100	5
Reduced Calorie (Weight Watchers)	1 Tbsp	40	5
Reduced Calorie, Cholesterol-Free (Weight Watchers)	1 Tbsp	40	none
Reduced Calorie Light Mayonnaise (Kraft)	1 Tbsp	45	5
Reduced Calorie, Light Mayonnaise, Hellmann's (CPC International, Inc)	1 Tbsp	50	10
Reduced Calorie, *Light N'Lively* (Kraft)	1 Tbsp	40	5
Reduced Calorie, Low Sodium (Weight Watchers)	1 Tbsp	40	5
Reduced Calorie Whipped Salad Dressing (Weight Watchers)	1 Tbsp	35	5

McDONALD'S

FOOD	PORTION SIZE	CALORIES	CHOLESTEROL (Mg)
Apple Danish	1	389	26
Apple Pie	1	253	12
Barbecue Sauce	2 Tbsp	60	<0.3
Big Mac	1	570	83
Biscuit w/Bacon, Egg, Cheese	1	483	263
Biscuit w/Biscuit Spread	1	330	9
Biscuit w/Sausage	1	467	48
Biscuit w/Sausage, Egg	1	585	285
Caramel Sundae	1	361	31
Cheese Danish, Iced	1	395	48
Cheeseburger	1	328	41
Cherry Pie	1	260	13
Chicken McNuggets	1	323	73

FOOD	PORTION SIZE	CALORIES	CHOLESTEROL (Mg)
Chocolate Chip Cookies	1	342	18
Chocolate Shake	1	383	30
Cinnamon Raisin Danish	1	445	35
English Muffin w/Butter	1	186	15
Filet O Fish	1	435	45
French Fries, reg	1	220	9
Hamburger	1	263	29
Hash Brown Potatoes	1	125	7
Honey	2 Tbsp	50	<0.1
Hot Cakes w/Butter, Syrup	1	500	47
Hot Fudge Sundae	1	357	27
Hot Mustard Sauce	2 Tbsp	63	3
Ice Cream, Soft Serve	1	189	24
Mc D.L.T.	1	680	101
McDonald Land Cookies	1	308	10
McMuffin Egg	1	340	259
McMuffin Sausage	1	427	59
McMuffin Sausage w/Egg	1	517	287
Quarter Pounder	1	427	81
Quarter Pounder w/Cheese	1	525	107
Salad, Chef	1	226	125
Salad, Shrimp	1	99	187
Salad, Garden	1	91	110
Salad, Chicken Oriental	1	146	92
Salad, Side	1	48	42
Salad Dressing, Bleu Cheese	1.25 oz	171	16
Salad Dressing, French	1 oz	114	<1
Salad Dressing, House	1 oz	163	7
Salad Dressing, Lite Vinaigrette	1 oz	25	<1
Salad Dressing, Oriental	1 oz	51	<1
Salad Dressing, 1000 Island	1.25 oz	198	24
Salad Topping, Bacon Bits	3 g	15	3
Salad Topping, Chow Mein	9 g	45	2
Salad Topping, Croutons	11g	52	<1

FOOD	PORTION SIZE	CALORIES	CHOLESTEROL (Mg)
Sausage, Pork	1	210	39
Scrambled Eggs	1	180	514
Strawberry Shake	1	362	32
Strawberry Sundae	1	320	25
Sweet & Sour Sauce	2 Tbsp	64	<0.1
Vanilla Shake	1	352	31

MEAT SUBSTITUTES
(*see also* FRANKFURTERS, HAM, LUNCHEON MEATS/COLD CUTS, SAUSAGE, TURKEY)

FOOD	PORTION SIZE	CALORIES	CHOLESTEROL (Mg)
Bolono (Worthington)	2 slices	70	none
Breakfast Links (Morningstar Farms)	1	49	none
Breakfast Patties (Morningstar Farms)	1	91	none
Breakfast Strips (Morningstar Farms)	3	85	none
Chicken Style Roll (Worthington)	2½ oz	170	none
Meatless Hotdog (Loma Linda)	1	101	none
Veg Skallops, canned (Worthington)	½ cup	70	none
Vegetarian Burger, canned (Worthington)	½ cup	160	none
Wham (Worthington)	3 slices	130	none

MILK
(*see also* MILK DRINKS, MILK FLAVORINGS)
The term regular refers to a whole milk product.

FOOD	PORTION SIZE	CALORIES	CHOLESTEROL (Mg)
Lowfat, 1% fat (Generic)	8 oz	102	10
Lowfat, 2% fat (Generic)	8 oz	122	20

FOOD	PORTION SIZE	CALORIES	CHOLESTEROL (Mg)
Lowfat, Buttermilk (Land O Lakes)	8 oz	100	10
Lowfat, buttermilk (Generic)	8 oz	98	10
Lowfat, Buttermilk Blend, Dry; Reconstituted (Saco)	1 cup (.8 oz dry)	79	5
Lowfat, Buttermilk 1.5% Fat (Friendship)	8 oz	120	13.6
Lowfat, Evaporated (Carnation)	½ cup	110	18
Lowfat, evaporated skim (Generic)	1 cup	200	10
Lowfat, Evaporated Skimmed (Carnation)	½ cup	100	5
Lowfat, protein fortified 1% fat (Generic)	8 oz	118	10
Lowfat, protein fortified 2% fat (Generic)	8 oz	138	20
Lowfat, skim (Generic)	8 oz	86	5
Lowfat, skim protein fortified (Generic)	8 oz	101	5
Nonfat Dry Mix 'N Drink, Instant (Saco)	8 oz	80	5
Nonfat Dry, Flash; reconstituted (Land O Lakes)	8 oz	80	5
Nonfat Dry, Instant (Carnation)	1 Tbsp	80	4
Nonfat dry, instantized (Generic)	⅓ cup	81	4
Nonfat dry, non instantized (Generic)	⅓ cup	145	8
Regular, coconut	½ cup	26	none
Regular, evaporated (Generic)	1 cup	327	71
Regular, Evaporated (Carnation)	½ cup	170	37
Regular, goat (Generic	8 oz	156	27
Regular, human	8 oz	172	34

FOOD	PORTION SIZE	CALORIES	CHOLESTEROL (Mg)
Regular, soybean milk (Generic)	8 oz	87	none
Regular, sweetened condensed (Generic)	1 cup	982	104
Regular, Sweetened Condensed, *Eagle* (Borden)	⅓ cup	320	35
Regular, whole, 3.3% fat (Generic)	8 oz	149	34
Regular, whole, 3.7% fat (Generic)	8 oz	156	34
Regular, whole, low sodium (Generic)	1 cup	149	34
Regular, whole dry (Generic)	⅓ cup	212	41

MILK DRINKS
(*see also* MILK, MILK FLAVORINGS)
All the following are ready-to-drink

Chocolate Milk (Land O Lakes)	8 oz	210	30
Chocolate milk, 1% fat (Generic)	8 oz	158	8
Chocolate Milk, 1% fat (Land O Lakes)	8 oz	160	5
Chocolate milk, 2% fat (Generic)	8 oz	180	18
Chocolate milk, whole, 3.3% fat (Generic)	8 oz	208	30
Chocolate Milk, Skim (Land O Lakes)	8 oz	140	5
Egg Nog (Generic)	8 oz	343	150
Egg Nog (Land O Lakes)	8 oz	300	123
Hot Cocoa; as prep w/whole milk (Generic)	8 oz	218	33

FOOD	PORTION SIZE	CALORIES	CHOLESTEROL (Mg)
Hot Cocoa, *70 Calorie Mix;* as prep w/water (Carnation)	8 oz	70	2
Hot Cocoa Sugar Free Mix; as prep w/water (Carnation)	8 oz	50	2
Hot Cocoa, *Swiss Miss,* Regular; as prep w/water (Beatrice)	8 oz	110	none
Malted milk, chocolate (Generic)	8 oz	233	34
Malted milk, natural flavor (Generic)	8 oz	236	37
Shake, fast food chocolate (Generic)	10 oz	360	37
Shake, fast food, strawberry (Generic)	10 oz	319	31
Shake, fast food, vanilla (Generic)	10 oz	314	32
Shake, thick, chocolate (Generic)	8 oz	290	24
Shake, thick, vanilla (Generic)	8 oz	273	29
Yoo-hoo	9 oz	150	none

MILK FLAVORINGS
(*see also* MILK, MILK DRINKS)

FOOD	PORTION SIZE	CALORIES	CHOLESTEROL (Mg)
Mix, Chocolate Flavor; as prep w/whole milk (Ovaltine)	1 cup	230	33
Mix, Chocolate Flavor, Malted, Instant (Horlicks)	1 Tbsp	85	2
Mix, Chocolate Flavor, *QUIK;* as prep w/whole milk (Nestle)	1 cup	240	33
Mix, chocolate malted (Generic)	1 Tbsp	28	tr

FOOD	PORTION SIZE	CALORIES	CHOLESTEROL (Mg)
Mix, cocoa, breakfast (Generic)	1 Tbsp	21	none
Mix, hot chocolate sweetened (Generic)	1 Tbsp	27	none
Mix, Instant (Hershey)	3½ oz	360	none
Mix, natural flavor, malted (Generic)	1 Tbsp	29	1
Mix, Natural Flavor, Malted Instant (Horlicks)	1 Tbsp	90	5
Mix, Natural, Malted Instant; as prep w/whole milk (Carnation)	1 cup	240	38
Mix, Natural Flavor, Malted, Non Instant (Horlicks)	1 Tbsp	117	none
Mix, Strawberry Flavor, *Quik;* as prep w/whole milk (Nestle)	1 cup	240	33
Syrup, Chocolate Flavored (Hershey)	1 Tbsp	37	none

MINERAL WATER

Bottled (Perrier)	6½ oz	0	none
Bottled (Poland Spring)	1 cup	0	none

MUFFINS
(*see* BREAD & ROLLS)

MUSTARD

Mustard, prepared (Kraft)	1 tsp	4	none

NON-DAIRY CREAMER
(*see* COFFEE WHITENERS)

FOOD	PORTION SIZE	CALORIES	CHOLESTEROL (Mg)

NOODLES & PASTA
(*see also* PIEROGI, POTATOES, SAUCES)

FOOD	PORTION SIZE	CALORIES	CHOLESTEROL (Mg)
Noodle, Egg; cooked (Muellers)	1 cup	210	63
Noodle, Egg; cooked (Ronzoni)	1 cup	220	80
Noodle, Egg Noodle w/Chicken Dinner; as prep (Kraft)	¾ cup	240	35
Noodle pudding (Generic)	½ cup	132	27
Noodles; cooked (Generic)	½ cup	100	25
Noodles, *Creamy Noodles 'n Tuna, Tuna Helper;* as prep	1 serving	282	20
Pasta, All Shapes; cooked (Muellers)	1 cup	210	none
Pasta, All Shapes; cooked (Prince)	1 cup	204	none
Pasta; cooked (Ronzoni)	1 cup	210	none
Pasta; cooked (San Giorgio)	1 cup	210	none
Pasta, Fettucini Alfredo (Home recipe)	1 cup	264	72
Pasta, Lasagna (Home recipe)	2½" sq	374	107
Pasta, Macaroni and Cheese Dinner; as prep (Kraft)	¾ cup	290	5
Pasta Meals Mini Lasagna in Sauce (Ragu)	7½ oz	170	none
Pasta Meals Shells In Sauce With Ground Beef (Ragu)	7½ oz	180	10
Pasta Meals Spaghetti In Sauce (Ragu)	7½ oz	160	none
Pasta primavera (Home recipe)	1 cup	358	66
Pasta, rigatoni w/sausage sauce (Home recipe)	¾ cup	260	59
Pasta, Spinach Linguini, *High Protein;* cooked (Buitoni)	1 cup	210	none
Pasta, *Superoni;* cooked (Prince)	1 cup	210	none

FOOD	PORTION SIZE	CALORIES	CHOLESTEROL (Mg)
Pasta, *Tangy Italian Style Spaghetti Dinner;* as prep (Kraft)	1 cup	310	5
Pasta w/meatballs & cheese (Home recipe)	1 cup	407	104
Pasta w/meatballs & tomato sauce (Home recipe)	1 cup	332	74
Pasta w/meatballs & tomato sauce, canned (Generic)	1 cup	258	123
Pasta w/tomato sauce & cheese canned (Generic)	1 cup	190	19

NUTRITIONAL SUPPLEMENTS

FOOD	PORTION SIZE	CALORIES	CHOLESTEROL (Mg)
Breakfast bar, chocolate chip (Generic)	1 bar	200	<1
Breakfast bar, chocolate crunch (Generic)	1 bar	190	<1
Breakfast bar, peanut butter crunch (Generic)	1 bar	190	<1
Breakfast bar, peanut butter crunch with chocolate chips (Generic)	1 bar	200	<1
Carnation Instant Breakfast, Vanilla	1 pkg	130	2
Carnation Instant Breakfast, Vanilla; as prep w/whole milk	1 cup	280	36
Carnation Slender Bar, Chocolate	2 bars	270	<1
Carnation Slender Bar, Chocolate Chip	2 bars	270	<1
Carnation Slender Bar, Chocolate Peanut Butter	2 bars	270	<1

FOOD	PORTION SIZE	CALORIES	CHOLESTEROL (Mg)
Carnation Slender Bar, Vanilla	2 bars	270	<1
Carnation Slender, canned, Banana	10 oz	220	5
Carnation Slender, canned, Chocolate	10 oz	220	4
Carnation Slender, canned, Chocolate Fudge	10 oz	220	4
Carnation Slender, canned, Chocolate Malt	10 oz	220	4
Carnation Slender, canned, Milk Chocolate	10 oz	220	4
Carnation Slender, canned, Peach	10 oz	220	5
Carnation Slender, canned, Strawberry	10 oz	220	5
Carnation Slender, canned, Vanilla	10 oz	220	5
Carnation Slender, instant, Chocolate	1 envelope	130	3
Carnation Slender, instant, Dutch chocolate	1 envelope	130	2
Carnation Slender, instant, Vanilla	1 envelope	130	3
NutriCare	1.13 oz serving	120	5
NutriCare; as prep w/2% milk	1 serving	260	25
NutriCare; as prep w/whole milk	1 serving	280	45
Sustacal Pudding	5 oz	240	<5

FOOD	PORTION SIZE	CALORIES	CHOLESTEROL (Mg)

NUTS
(*See also* COCONUT, PEANUT BUTTER)

FOOD	PORTION SIZE	CALORIES	CHOLESTEROL (Mg)
Almond paste (Generic)	1 oz	127	none
Almonds, Whole Sliced (Planters)	1 oz	170	none
Cashew butter (Generic)	1 Tbsp	94	none
Chestnuts; roasted & shelled (Generic)	½ cup	175	none
Macadamia nuts (Generic)	½ cup	470	none
Peanuts, *Dry Roasted* (Planters)	1 oz	160	none
Peanuts, *Honey Roast* (Planters)	1 oz	170	none
Pecans (Generic)	1 oz	190	none
Pine nuts (pignolia) (Generic)	1 oz	146	none
Pistachio nuts (Generic)	½ cup	369	none
Tahini, sesame butter (Generic)	1 Tbsp	86	none
Walnuts, English (Planters)	1 oz	190	none

OILS
(*see also* BUTTER, FATS, MARGARINE, MAYONNAISE)

FOOD	PORTION SIZE	CALORIES	CHOLESTEROL (Mg)
Corn (generic)	1 Tbsp	120	none
Cottonseed (Generic)	1 Tbsp	120	none
Crisco	1 Tbsp	124	none
Mazola No-Stick spray	2 second spray	8	none
Olive (Generic)	1 Tbsp	119	none
PAM	1 spray (1.3 g)	2	none
Peanut (Generic)	1 Tbsp	119	none
Puritan (Procter & Gamble)	1 Tbsp	119	none
Safflower (Generic)	1 Tbsp	120	none

FOOD	PORTION SIZE	CALORIES	CHOLESTEROL (Mg)
Soybean (Generic)	1 Tbsp	120	none
Sunflower (Generic)	1 Tbsp	120	none
Wesson	1 Tbsp	120	none

The following oils are used as nutrient supplements, not as foods

FOOD	PORTION SIZE	CALORIES	CHOLESTEROL (Mg)
Cod liver oil	1 Tbsp	120	85
Omega-3, fish oils	650 mg capsule	14	5

OLIVES

FOOD	PORTION SIZE	CALORIES	CHOLESTEROL (Mg)
Black ripe, canned (Generic)	13 jumbo	80	none
Black ripe, canned (Generic)	12 med	56	none
Greek (Generic)	3 med	64	none
Green (Generic)	2 med	15	none

ORGAN MEATS
(*see* BRAINS, GIBLETS, GIZZARD, HEART, KIDNEY, LIVER, SWEETBREAD)

PANCAKES/HOT CAKES
(*see also* CREPES, FRENCH TOAST, WAFFLES)

FOOD	PORTION SIZE	CALORIES	CHOLESTEROL (Mg)
Hot Cakes w/Butter & Syrup (McDonald's)	1 portion	500	47
Pancake (Home recipe)	4" diam	61	20
Pancake & sausage, w/o syrup & butter (Generic)	1 portion	407	77
Pancake & Waffle Mix *Hungry Jack Extra Lights;* as prep (Pillsbury)	3 pancakes 4" diam	210	150

FOOD	PORTION SIZE	CALORIES	CHOLESTEROL (Mg)
Pancake & Waffle Original Mix, *Aunt Jemima;* as prep (Quaker)	3 pancakes 4″ diam	200	146
Pancake Platter w/Syrup, Butter (Roy Rogers)	1 portion	452	53
Pancake Platter w/Syrup, Butter, Bacon (Roy Rogers)	1 portion	493	63
Pancake Platter w/Syrup, Butter, Ham (Roy Rogers)	1 portion	506	73
Pancake Platter w/Syrup, Butter, Sausage (Roy Rogers)	1 portion	608	94
Pancake, plain (Home recipe)	4″ diam	61	20
Pancake, buttermilk (Home recipe)	4″ diam	61	20
Pancake, From Batter (Mrs. Smith's)	3 medium	230	40
Pancakes w/o Butter & Syrup (Whataburger)	1 portion	199	34

PEANUT BUTTER
(*see also* BUTTER, NUTS)

FOOD	PORTION SIZE	CALORIES	CHOLESTEROL (Mg)
Peanut butter (Generic)	1 Tbsp	86	none
Jif, chunky	2 Tbsp	186	none
Jif, creamy	2 Tbsp	186	none
Skippy	1 Tbsp	95	none

PASTA
(*see* NOODLES & PASTA)

PÂTÉ
(*see* LIVER)

FOOD	PORTION SIZE	CALORIES	CHOLESTEROL (Mg)

PICKLE

Butter & butter	4 slices	18	none
Chutney, tomato	1 Tbsp	41	none
Dill	1 med	11	none
Sweet Gherkin	1 sm	22	none

PIE CRUST

(*see also* PIE)

Frozen (Pet Ritz)	⅛ crust	107	8
Frozen (Generic)	1⁄16 crust	130	6

PIE

(*see also* CAKE, COOKIES, DOUGHNUTS, PIE CRUST, QUICHE)

Apple Lattice, frzn (Mrs. Smith)	⅛ of 9 ⅝″ pie	350	5
Apple (Home recipe)	⅐ of 9″ pie	402	7
Apple, frzn (Mrs. Smith's)	⅛ of 9 ⅝″ pie	390	10
Apple *Natural Juice,* frzn (Mrs. Smith)	⅐ of 9″ pie	420	5
Apple, *Old Fashioned,* frzn (Mrs. Smith)	⅛ of 9 ⅝″ pie	515	10
Apple Streusel, frzn (Mrs. Smith)	⅐ of 9″ pie	420	5
Banana Cream (Home recipe)	⅐ of 9″ pie	354	83
Banana Cream, frzn (Mrs. Smith)	⅛ of 9 ⅝″ pie	240	5
Blackberry (Home recipe)	⅐ of 9″ pie	372	4
Blueberry (Home recipe)	⅐ of 9″ pie	411	4
Blueberry (Hostess)	1 pie	390	18
Blueberry, frzn (Mrs. Smith)	⅛ of 9 ⅝″ pie	380	10
Boston Cream (Mrs. Smith)	⅛ of 9 ⅝″ pie	260	20

FOOD	PORTION SIZE	CALORIES	CHOLESTEROL (Mg)
Butterscotch (Home recipe)	⅐ of 9″ pie	417	108
Cherry (Home recipe)	⅐ of 9″ pie	462	8
Cherry (Hostess)	1 pie	390	18
Cherry, frzn (Mrs. Smith)	⅛ of 9 ⅝″ pie	350	5
Cherry, *Natural Juice,* frzn (Mrs. Smith)	⅐ of 9″ pie	410	10
Chess (Home recipe)	⅐ of 9″ pie	682	201
Chocolate chiffon (Home recipe)	⅐ of 9″ pie	337	94
Chocolate Cream, frzn (Mrs. Smith)	⅛ of 9 ⅝″ pie	270	5
Chocolate meringue (Home recipe)	⅐ of 9″ pie	371	83
Chocolate Mousse; as prep w/ whole milk (Jell-O)	⅛ of pie from mix	250	30
Coconut Cream, frzn (Mrs. Smith)	⅛ of 9 ⅝″ pie	270	5
Coconut Cream; as prep w/ whole milk (Jell-O)	⅛ of 9 ⅝″ pie	260	30
Coconut custard (Home recipe)	⅐ of 9″ pie	346	78
Coconut Custard, frzn (Mrs. Smith)	⅛ of 9 ⅝″ pie	330	50
Custard (Home recipe)	⅐ of 9″ pie	324	136
Custard, frzn (Mrs. Smith)	⅛ of 9 ⅝″ pie	300	65
Grasshopper (Home recipe)	⅐ of 9″ pie	396	179
Key lime (Home recipe)	⅐ of 9″ pie	393	87
Lemon chiffon (Home recipe)	⅐ of 9″ pie	381	145
Lemon Cream, frzn (Mrs. Smith)	⅛ of 9 ⅝″ pie	245	5
Lemon meringue (Home recipe)	⅐ of 9″ pie	399	91
Lemon Meringue, frzn (Mrs. Smith)	⅛ of 9 ⅝″ pie	310	35
Lemon (Jell-O)	⅙ of 9″ pie from mix	170	90

FOOD	PORTION SIZE	CALORIES	CHOLESTEROL (Mg)
Mince (Home recipe)	1/7 of 9″ pie	441	6
Peach (Mrs. Smith)	1/8 of 9 5/8″ pie	365	10
Pecan (Home recipe)	1/7 of 9″ pie	566	114
Pecan, frzn (Mrs. Smith)	1/8 of 9 5/8″ pie	510	30
Pineapple chiffon (Generic)	1/7 of 9″ pie	337	20
Pumpkin (Home recipe)	1/7 of 9″ pie	287	84
Pumpkin Custard (Mrs. Smith)	1/8 of 9 5/8″ pie	310	30
Raisin (Home recipe)	1/7 of 9″ pie	545	132
Rhubarb (Home recipe)	1/7 of 9″ pie	414	7
Squash (Home recipe)	1/7 of 9″ pie	311	67
Strawberry (Home recipe)	1/7 of 9″ pie	282	none

PIEROGI

(*see also* NOODLES & PASTA, POTATOES)

Pierogi (Home recipe)	3/4 cup	307	49

PIGS EARS & FEET

(*see* PORK)

PIZZA

(*see also* DOMINO'S PIZZA)

W/cheese	1/7 of 10″ pie (2 oz)	140	23
W/cheese & sausage	1/8 of 14″ pie (3½ oz)	266	35

FOOD	PORTION SIZE	CALORIES	CHOLESTEROL (Mg)

PORK
(*see also* BACON, HAM, LUNCHEON MEATS/COLD CUTS, SAUSAGE)

FOOD	PORTION SIZE	CALORIES	CHOLESTEROL (Mg)
Blade steak, w/o bone, fully trimmed; cooked	3 oz	207	75
Blade steak; w/o bone, not trimmed; cooked	3 oz	300	76
Bologna (Generic)	1 slice (1 oz)	70	17
Boston butt, w/o bone, fully trimmed; roasted	3 slices (3 oz)	207	75
Boston butt, w/o bone, not trimmed; roasted	3 slices (3 oz)	300	76
Braunschweiger, liver sausage (Generic)	1 oz	102	44
Breakfast strips; cooked (Generic)	3 slices (34 g)	156	36
Chitterlings; cooked (Home recipe)	3 oz	258	122
Ears; cooked (Home recipe)	1 (3 oz)	183	99
Feet; boiled (Generic)	1	140	77
Fritter (Home recipe)	¾ cup (6 oz)	487	222
Ham fresh, leg center, w/o bone, fully trimmed; cooked	1 slice (3 oz)	184	75
Ham fresh, leg center, w/o bone, not trimmed; cooked	1 slice (3 oz)	318	76
Ham fresh, leg, fully trimmed; roasted	2 slices (3 oz)	184	75
Ham fresh, leg, fully trimmed; roasted, chopped	½ cup	152	62
Ham fresh, leg, not trimmed; roasted	2 slices (3 oz)	318	76

FOOD	PORTION SIZE	CALORIES	CHOLESTEROL (Mg)
Ham fresh, leg, not trimmed; roasted, chopped	½ cup	262	62
Ham fresh, loin, fully trimmed; roasted	½ cup	178	62
Liver cheese (Generic)	1 oz	86	49
Liver; braised	3 oz	141	302
Liverwurst (Generic)	1 oz	92	45
Loin chop, w/bone, fully trimmed; broiled	3 oz	227	74
Loin chop, w/bone, not trimmed; broiled	4 oz	454	103
Loin chop, w/o bone, fully trimmed; broiled	3 oz	229	75
Loin chop, w/o bone, not trimmed; broiled	3 oz	332	76
Loin roast, w/o bone, fully trimmed; roasted	3 slices (3 oz)	216	75
Loin roast, w/o bone, fully trimmed; cooked, ground	½ cup	140	48
Loin roast, w/o bone, fully trimmed; cooked, chopped	½ cup	178	62
Loin roast, w/o bone, not trimmed; cooked, ground	½ cup	199	49
Loin roast, w/o bone, not trimmed; cooked, chopped	½ cup	253	62
Luncheon meat, canned (Generic)	1 oz	95	18
Meat, not trimmed; cooked, cubed	½ cup	261	62
Meat, not trimmed; cooked, ground	½ cup	205	49
Pancreas; braised	3 oz	186	268
Patty (Home recipe)	3″ diam	306	73

FOOD	PORTION SIZE	CALORIES	CHOLESTEROL (Mg)
Picnic, smoked, w/o bone, fully trimmed	3 slices (3 oz)	179	75
Picnic, smoked, w/o bone, not trimmed	3 slices (3 oz)	275	76
Picnic, w/o bone, fully trimmed; roasted	3 slices (3 oz)	180	75
Picnic, w/o bone, not trimmed; roasted	3 slices (3 oz)	318	76
Rib chop, w/bone, fully trimmed; broiled	3 oz	227	74
Rib chop, w/bone, not trimmed; broiled	4 oz	454	103
Rib chop, w/o bone, fully trimmed; broiled	3 oz	229	75
Rib chop, w/o bone, not trimmed; broiled	3 oz	332	76
Spam (Hormel)	1 oz	88	25
Spare ribs, fully trimmed; cooked	4" rib	66	14
Spare ribs, fully trimmed; cooked	5" rib	82	18
Spare ribs, fully trimmed; cooked	6" rib	103	22
Spare ribs, not trimmed; cooked	6" rib	110	22
Spare ribs, not trimmed; cooked	5" rib	88	18
Spare ribs, not trimmed; cooked	4" rib	70	14
Spleen; braised	3 oz	127	428
Tail; simmered	3 oz	336	110
Tongue; braised	3 oz	230	124

FOOD	PORTION SIZE	CALORIES	CHOLESTEROL (Mg)

POT PIE
(*see also* BEEF, CHICKEN)

FOOD	PORTION SIZE	CALORIES	CHOLESTEROL (Mg)
Vegetarian, frzn (Worthington)	8 oz	450	none

POTATOES
(*see also* NOODLES & PASTA, PIEROGI)

FOOD	PORTION SIZE	CALORIES	CHOLESTEROL (Mg)
Baked	1 med	95	none
Boiled, w/skin	1 med	76	none
Cottage fries, frzn (Generic)	⅔ cup	116	none
French fries; as prep from fresh (Home recipe)	½ cup	151	tr
French Fries, frzn (Bird's Eye)	¾ cup	136	none
French Fries, frzn; oven heated (Generic)	½ cup	121	none
Hash Browns, frzn (Bird's Eye)	¾ cup	72	none
Hash Browns; as prep w/ vegetable shortening (Home recipe)	½ cup	177	tr
Mashed, *French's Idaho;* as prep (Pillsbury)	½ cup	130	12
Mashed, *Hungry Jack;* as prep (Pillsbury)	½ cup	130	17
Mashed, plain (Home recipe)	½ cup	67	none
Mashed, *Potato Buds;* as prep (Betty Crocker)	½ cup	130	17
Potato au Gratin w/cheese (Generic)	½ cup	178	18
Potato Pancakes; as prep (Frenchs)	1	80	10
Potato Puffs, frzn (Bird's Eye)	½ cup	192	32
Salad, potato w/mayonnaise (Home recipe)	½ cup	145	65

FOOD	PORTION SIZE	CALORIES	CHOLESTEROL (Mg)
Scalloped (Home recipe)	½ cup	127	7
Tiny Taters, frzn (Bird's Eye)	⅔ cup	203	none
Triangles, frzn (Bird's Eye)	2 patties	143	none
Wedges, Farm Style, frzn (Bird's Eye)	3 oz	107	none

PUDDING
(*see also* PUDDING POPS)

FOOD	PORTION SIZE	CALORIES	CHOLESTEROL (Mg)
Banana, Instant, Sugar Free; as prep w/2% milk (Jell-O)	½ cup	90	10
Banana Cream; as prep w/skim milk (Jell-O)	½ cup	123	2
Banana Cream; as prep w/ whole milk (Jell-O)	½ cup	155	17
Banana cream, instant; as prep w/whole milk (Generic)	½ cup	172	17
Banana Cream, Instant; as prep w/whole milk (Jell-O)	½ cup	160	15
Bread, w/raisins (Home recipe)	½ cup	180	77
Butter pecan, instant; as prep w/whole milk (Generic)	½ cup	174	17
Butter Pecan, Instant; as prep w/whole milk (Jell-O)	½ cup	170	15
Butterscotch; as prep w/skim milk (Generic)	½ cup	136	2
Butterscotch; as prep w/whole milk (Generic)	½ cup	169	17
Butterscotch; as prep w/whole milk (Jell-O)	½ cup	170	15
Butterscotch, Instant; as prep w/whole milk (Jell-O)	½ cup	160	15

FOOD	PORTION SIZE	CALORIES	CHOLESTEROL (Mg)
Butterscotch, Instant, Sugar Free; as prep w/2% milk (Jell-O)	½ cup	90	10
Butterscotch, Reduced Calorie; as prep w/skim milk (D-zerta)	½ cup	69	2
Chocolate (Generic)	1 pkg	404	none
Chocolate; as prep w/whole milk (Jell-O)	½ cup	160	15
Chocolate, instant; as prep w/ whole milk (Generic)	½ cup	179	17
Chocolate, Instant (Jell-O)	1 pkg	725	tr
Chocolate, Instant; as prep w/ whole milk (Jell-O)	½ cup	180	17
Chocolate, Reduced Calorie; as prep w/skim milk (D-zerta)	½ cup	60	2
Chocolate, *Rich & Luscious Mousse;* as prep w/whole milk (Jell-O)	½ cup	150	10
Chocolate, Instant, Sugar Free; as prep w/2% milk (Jell-O)	½ cup	100	10
Chocolate, Sugar Free; as prep w/2% milk (Jell-O)	½ cup	90	10
Chocolate Fudge; as prep w/ whole milk (Jell-O)	½ cup	160	15
Chocolate fudge, instant mix; as prep w/whole milk (Generic)	½ cup	178	17
Chocolate Fudge, Instant; as prep w/whole milk (Jell-O)	½ cup	180	15
Chocolate Fudge, Instant, Sugar Free; as prep w/2% milk (Jell-O)	½ cup	100	10

FOOD	PORTION SIZE	CALORIES	CHOLESTEROL (Mg)
Chocolate Fudge, *Rich & Luscious Mousse;* as prep w/whole milk (Jell-O)	½ cup	150	10
Coconut cream, instant; as prep w/whole milk (Generic)	½ cup	184	17
Coconut Cream, Instant; as prep w/whole milk (Jell-O)	½ cup	180	15
Custard Mix, Golden Egg, *Americana;* as prep w/whole milk (Jell-O)	½ cup	160	80
French Vanilla; as prep w/whole milk (Jell-O)	½ cup	170	15
French vanilla, instant; as prep w/whole milk (Generic)	½ cup	172	17
French Vanilla, Instant; as prep w/whole milk (Jell-O)	½ cup	160	15
Lemon, instant mix; as prep w/whole milk (Generic)	½ cup	178	17
Lemon, Instant; as prep w/whole milk (Jell-O)	½ cup	170	15
Milk Chocolate; as prep w/whole milk (Jell-O)	½ cup	160	15
Milk Chocolate, Instant; as prep w/whole milk (Jell-O)	½ cup	180	15
Pineapple cream, instant; as prep w/whole milk (Generic)	½ cup	172	17
Pineapple Cream, Instant; as prep w/whole milk (Jell-O)	½ cup	160	15
Pistachio, instant; as prep w/whole milk (Generic)	½ cup	182	17
Pistachio, Instant; as prep w/whole milk (Jell-O)	½ cup	170	15
Pistachio, Instant, Sugar free, as prep w/2% milk (Jell-O)	½ cup	100	10

FOOD	PORTION SIZE	CALORIES	CHOLESTEROL (Mg)
Pumpkin (Home recipe)	½ cup	170	105
Rice; as prep w/whole milk (Generic)	½ cup	175	17
Rice, *Americana;* as prep w/ whole milk (Jell-O)	½ cup	170	15
Rice w/raisins (Home recipe)	½ cup	246	136
Tapioca; as prep w/whole milk (Generic)	½ cup	160	17
Tapioca, Chocolate, *Americana;* as prep w/whole milk (Jell-O)	½ cup	170	15
Tapioca cream (Home recipe)	½ cup	169	111
Tapioca, Vanilla, *Americana;* as prep w/whole milk (Jell-O)	½ cup	160	15
Tomato (Home recipe)	½ cup	212	21
Vanilla, Cool 'N Creamy (Bird's Eye)	½ cup	173	17
Vanilla; as prep w/skim milk (Jell-O)	½ cup	124	2
Vanilla; as prep w/whole milk (Jell-O)	½ cup	160	15
Vanilla, Instant; as prep w/ whole milk (Jell-O)	½ cup	170	15
Vanilla, Instant; Sugar Free; as prep w/2% milk (Jell-O)	½ cup	90	10
Vanilla, Reduced Calorie; as prep w/skim milk (D-Zerta)	½ cup	70	2
Vanilla, Sugar Free; as prep w/2% milk (Jell-O)	½ cup	80	10

FOOD	PORTION SIZE	CALORIES	CHOLESTEROL (Mg)

PUDDING POP
(see also ICE CREAM & FROZEN DESSERTS, PUDDING)

Banana (Generic)	1 pop	94	1
Butterscotch (Generic)	1 pop	94	1
Chocolate (Jell-O)	1 pop	80	none
Chocolate, Carmel Swirl (Jell-O)	1 pop	80	none
Chocolate, Chocolate Covered (Jell-O)	1 pop	130	none
Chocolate fudge (Generic)	1 pop	99	1
Chocolate Vanilla Swirl (Jell-O)	1 pop	70	none
Chocolate w/Chocolate Chip (Jell-O)	1 pop	80	none
Vanilla (Jell-O)	1 pop	70	none
Vanilla, Chocolate Covered (Jell-O)	1 pop	130	none
Vanilla, w/Chocolate Chips (Jell-O)	1 pop	80	none

QUICHE
(see also CAKE, COOKIES, DOUGHNUTS, PIE)

Florentine, frzn (Mrs. Smith's)	9½ oz	625	70
Lorraine (Home recipe)	⅙ of 9" pie	379	159
Lorraine (Mrs. Smith's)	9½ oz	720	95
Mushroom, frzn (Mrs. Smith's)	9½ oz	595	75

RED LOBSTER

Values given below are for raw portions. The method of preparation may add additional calories and/or cholesterol.

Atlantic Cod	5 oz	100	70
Atlantic Ocean Perch	5 oz	130	75
Blacktip Shark	5 oz	150	60

FOOD	PORTION SIZE	CALORIES	CHOLESTEROL (Mg)
Calico Scallops	5 oz	180	115
Catfish	5 oz	170	85
Cherrystone Clams	5 oz	130	80
Chicken Breast	4 oz	120	65
Deep Sea Scallops	5 oz	130	50
Flounder	5 oz	100	70
Grouper	5 oz	110	65
Haddock	5 oz	110	85
Halibut	5 oz	110	60
Hamburger	⅓ lb	320	105
King Crab Legs	1 lb	170	100
Langostino	5 oz	120	210
Lemon Sole	5 oz	120	65
Mackerel	5 oz	190	100
Maine Lobster	1¼ lb	240	310
Mako Shark	5 oz	140	100
Monkfish	5 oz	110	80
Mussels	3 oz	70	50
Norwegian Salmon	5 oz	230	80
Oysters, Raw On Half Shell	6 med	110	60
Pollock	5 oz	120	90
Porterhouse Steak	18 oz	1420	290
Rainbow Trout	5 oz	170	90
Red Rockfish	5 oz	90	85
Red Snapper	5 oz	110	70
Rock Lobster	1 tail (5 oz)	230	200
Shrimp	5 oz	120	230
Sirloin Steak	7 oz	570	140
Snow Crab Legs	1 lb	150	130
Sockeye Salmon	5 oz	160	50
Strip Steak	7 oz	690	140
Swordfish	5 oz	100	100
Tilefish	5 oz	100	80
Yellowfin Tuna	5 oz	180	70

FOOD	PORTION SIZE	CALORIES	CHOLESTEROL (Mg)

RICE

FOOD	PORTION SIZE	CALORIES	CHOLESTEROL (Mg)
Beef Flavored, Instant; cooked (Minute Rice)	½ cup	152	10
Beef Flavour'd; cooked (Uncle Ben's)	½ cup	103	none
Brown Rice; cooked (Uncle Ben's)	½ cup	100	none
Brown rice, long grain; cooked (Generic)	½ cup	104	none
Brown Rice, Natural Long Grain; cooked (Mahatma)	1 cup	220	none
Chicken Flavored; cooked (Uncle Ben's)	½ cup	100	tr
Chicken Flavored, Instant; cooked (Minute Rice)	½ cup	153	10
Chicken, *Rice-A-Roni;* cooked (Golden Grain)	¾ cup	196	11
Chinese Fried, Instant; cooked (Minute Rice)	½ cup	159	none
Chinese style, fried rice (Home recipe)	¾ cup	140	none
Curried; cooked (Uncle Ben's)	½ cup	100	none
Drumstick Rice Mix; as prep w/ butter (Minute Rice)	½ cup	150	10
Italian Style, Northern, frzn; cooked (Bird's Eye)	½ cup	111	3
Oriental style; cooked (Bird's Eye)	½ cup	125	none
Pilaf (Home recipe)	½ cup	84	22
Rib Roast; as prep w/butter (Minute Rice)	½ cup	150	10
Spanish; cooked (Uncle Ben's)	½ cup	109	none
Spanish, Instant; cooked (Minute Rice)	½ cup	150	10

FOOD	PORTION SIZE	CALORIES	CHOLESTEROL (Mg)
Spanish Style, frzn; cooked (Bird's Eye)	½ cup	124	none
Spanish tomato rice (Home recipe)	¾ cup	363	35
Spanish, w/Butter & Tomatoes *Rice-A-Roni;* cooked (Golden Grain)	¾ cup	172	11
Tuna, Creamy Rice'n, *Tuna Helper;* as prep	1 serving	252	20
White, Converted; cooked (Uncle Ben's)	½ cup	91	none
White, enriched long grain; cooked (Generic)	½ cup	112	none
White, Enriched, Long Grain; cooked (Mahatma)	1 cup	200	none
White, Extra Long Grained, Enriched; cooked (Carolina)	½ cup	100	none
White, Long Grain & Wild Rice; as prep w/butter (Minute Rice)	½ cup	150	10
White, Long Grained & Wild Rice, Instant; cooked (Minute Rice)	½ cup	147	10
White, *Minute Rice;* cooked (General Foods)	1 cup	180	none
White, Quick; cooked (Uncle Ben's)	½ cup	79	none

ROY ROGERS

Apple Danish	1	249	15
Bacon Cheeseburger	1	581	103
Biscuit	1	231	5
Breakfast Crescent Sandwich	1	401	148

FOOD	PORTION SIZE	CALORIES	CHOLESTEROL (Mg)
Breakfast Crescent Sandwich w/Bacon	1	431	156
Breakfast Crescent Sandwich w/Ham	1	557	189
Breakfast Crescent Sandwich w/Sausage	1	449	168
Brownie	1	264	10
Caramel Sundae	1	293	23
Cheese Danish	1	254	11
Cheeseburger	1	563	95
Cherry Danish	1	271	11
Chicken Breast	1	412	118
Chicken, Breast & Wing	1	604	165
Chicken, Drumstick/Leg	1	140	40
Chicken Nuggets	6	267	51
Chicken, Thigh	1	296	85
Chicken, Thigh & Leg	1	436	125
Chicken, Wing	1	192	47
Chocolate Shake	1	358	37
Cole Slaw	1	110	5
Crescent Roll	1	287	5
Egg & Biscuit Platter	1	394	284
Egg & Biscuit Platter w/Bacon	1	435	294
Egg & Biscuit Platter w/Ham	1	442	304
Egg & Biscuit Platter w/ Sausage	1	550	325
French Fries, lg	1	357	56
French Fries, reg	1	268	42
Hamburger	1	456	73
Hot Chocolate	6 oz	123	35
Hot Fudge Sundae	1	337	23
Hot Topped Potato Plain	1	211	none
Hot Topped Potato w/Bacon 'N Cheese	1	397	34

FOOD	PORTION SIZE	CALORIES	CHOLESTEROL (Mg)
Hot Topped Potato w/Broccoli 'N Cheese	1	376	19
Hot Topped Potato w/Oleo	1	274	none
Hot Topped Potato w/Sour Cream & Chives	1	408	31
Hot Topped Potato w/Taco Beef 'N Cheese	1	463	37
Macaroni Salad	1	186	5
Milk	8 oz	150	33
Orange Juice	7 oz	99	none
Pancake Platter w/Syrup, Butter	1	452	53
Pancake Platter w/Syrup, Butter, Bacon	1	493	63
Pancake Platter w/Syrup, Butter, Ham	1	506	73
Pancake Platter w/Syrup, Butter, Sausage	1	608	94
Potato Salad	1	107	5
Roast Beef, lg	1	360	73
Roast Beef w/Cheese, lg	1	467	95
Roast Beef Sandwich	1	317	55
Roast Beef Sandwich w/Cheese	1	424	77
RR Bar Burger	1	611	115
Strawberry Shake	1	315	37
Strawberry Shortcake	1	447	28
Strawberry Sundae	1	216	23
Vanilla Shake	1	306	40

FOOD	PORTION SIZE	CALORIES	CHOLESTEROL (Mg)

SALADS

Chef (Home recipe)	1½ cups	386	244
Cole Slaw (Kentucky Fried Chicken)	1 portion	103	4
Cole Slaw (Roy Rogers)	1 portion	110	5
Cole Slaw (Long John Silver's)	1 portion	182	12
Cole slaw (Generic)	½ cup	42	5
Popeye (Home recipe)	½ cup	204	75
Potato Salad (Roy Rogers)	1 portion	107	5
Potato Salad (Kentucky Fried Chicken)	1 portion	141	11
Three bean (Home recipe)	¾ cup	230	none
Tossed (Home recipe)	1 cup	32	none
Tuna salad (Home recipe)	½ cup	188	40
Waldorf (Home recipe)	½ cup	79	8.

SALAD DRESSINGS

(*see also* DIPS; GRAVY; SAUCES; SOUPS, DRY)

All values below are given for salad dressings prepared according to package directions. Many salad dressings contain a very small amount of cholesterol in a one tablespoon portion. Some manufacturers' laboratory analysis information on cholesterol consider amounts less than 5 mg. in a serving as either none or trace (tr). If you use portions larger than those shown below, you may be getting a few milligrams of cholesterol.

Bacon & Buttermilk (Kraft)	1 Tbsp	80	none
Bacon & Tomato (Kraft)	1 Tbsp	70	none
Bacon & Tomato, Reduced Calorie (Kraft)	1 Tbsp	30	none
Bacon, Creamy, Reduced Calorie (Kraft)	1 Tbsp	30	none

FOOD	PORTION SIZE	CALORIES	CHOLESTEROL (Mg)
Bleu Cheese & Herbs; as prep (Good Seasons)	1 Tbsp	80	none
Blue Bright Day (United Food Industries)	1 Tbsp	60	none
Blue Cheese, Chunky (Kraft)	1 Tbsp	70	none
Blue Cheese, Chunky, *Wish-Bone Lite* (Lipton)	1 Tbsp	40	none
Blue Cheese, Chunky, Reduced Calorie (Kraft)	1 Tbsp	30	none
Blue Cheese, Reduced Calorie, *Roka Brand* (Kraft)	1 Tbsp	14	5
Blue Cheese & Bacon, *Philadelphia Brand* (Kraft)	1 Tbsp	70	none
Buttermilk, *Wish-Bone Lite* (Lipton)	1 Tbsp	50	none
Buttermilk, Creamy (Kraft)	1 Tbsp	80	5
Buttermilk, Creamy, Reduced Calorie (Kraft)	1 Tbsp	30	none
Buttermilk, Farm Style; as prep (Good Seasons)	1 Tbsp	60	5
Buttermilk & Chives, Creamy (Kraft)	1 Tbsp	80	5
Caesar, *Golden* (Kraft)	1 Tbsp	70	none
Caesar, *Wish-Bone* (Lipton)	1 Tbsp	70	none
Cheddar & Bacon, *Wish-Bone* (Lipton)	1 Tbsp	70	none
Cheese, *Roka Brand* (Kraft)	1 Tbsp	60	10
Cheese Garlic; as prep (Good Seasons)	1 Tbsp	80	none
Coleslaw Dressing (Kraft)	1 Tbsp	70	10
Cucumber, Creamy (Kraft)	1 Tbsp	70	none
Cucumber, Creamy, *Wish-Bone* (Lipton)	1 Tbsp	80	none

FOOD	PORTION SIZE	CALORIES	CHOLESTEROL (Mg)
Cucumber, Creamy, *Wish-Bone Lite* (Lipton)	1 Tbsp	40	none
Cucumber, Creamy, Reduced Calorie (Kraft)	1 Tbsp	30	none
French (Kraft)	1 Tbsp	60	none
French, Catalina (Kraft)	1 Tbsp	70	none
French, Deluxe, *Wish-Bone* (Lipton)	1 Tbsp	50	none
French, Garlic, *Wish-Bone* (Lipton)	1 Tbsp	60	none
French, Herbal, *Wish-Bone* (Lipton)	1 Tbsp	60	none
French, Lite-Line, *Wish-Bone* (Lipton)	1 Tbsp	30	none
French, Reduced Calorie (Kraft)	1 Tbsp	25	none
French, Sweet N' Spicy, *Wish-Bone* (Lipton)	1 Tbsp	70	none
Garlic, Creamy, *Wish-Bone* (Lipton)	1 Tbsp	80	none
Garlic & Chives, *Philadelphia Brand* (Kraft)	1 Tbsp	70	none
Garlic & Herbs; as prep (Good Seasons)	1 Tbsp	80	none
Herb, Classic; as prep (Good Seasons)	1 Tbsp	80	none
Italian; as prep (Good Seasons)	1 Tbsp	80	none
Italian, *Wish-Bone* (Lipton)	1 Tbsp	70	none
Italian, *Wish-Bone Lite* (Lipton)	1 Tbsp	30	none
Italian, Cheese; as prep (Good Seasons)	1 Tbsp	80	none
Italian, Creamy, *Wish-Bone* (Lipton)	1 Tbsp	60	none
Italian, Creamy, *Wish-Bone Lite* (Lipton)	1 Tbsp	30	none

FOOD	PORTION SIZE	CALORIES	CHOLESTEROL (Mg)
Italian, Creamy (Weight Watchers)	1 Tbsp	50	5
Italian, Creamy, Reduced Calorie (Kraft)	1 Tbsp	25	none
Italian, Creamy, w/Real Sour Cream (Kraft)	1 Tbsp	60	none
Italian, Herb, *Philadelphia Brand* (Kraft)	1 Tbsp	70	none
Italian, Herbal, *Wish-Bone* (Lipton)	1 Tbsp	70	none
Italian, Lite; as prep (Good Seasons)	1 Tbsp	25	none
Italian, Mild; as prep (Good Seasons)	1 Tbsp	90	none
Italian, No Oil; as prep (Good Seasons)	1 Tbsp	6	none
Italian, Oil-Free (Kraft)	1 Tbsp	4	none
Italian, Reduced Calorie (Kraft)	1 Tbsp	6	none
Italian, Robusto, *Wish-Bone* (Lipton)	1 Tbsp	80	none
Italian, Zesty; as prep (Good Seasons)	1 Tbsp	80	none
Italian, Zesty (Kraft)	1 Tbsp	70	none
Italian, Zesty Lite; as prep (Good Seasons)	1 Tbsp	25	none
Lemon & Herbs; as prep (Good Seasons)	1 Tbsp	80	none
Oil & Vinegar (Home recipe)	1 Tbsp	70	none
Oil & Vinegar (Kraft)	1 Tbsp	70	none
Onion & Chive, *Wish-Bone Lite* (Lipton)	1 Tbsp	40	none
Onion & Chives, Creamy (Kraft)	1 Tbsp	70	none
Russian (Kraft)	1 Tbsp	60	none
Russian, *Wish-Bone* (Lipton)	1 Tbsp	45	none

FOOD	PORTION SIZE	CALORIES	CHOLESTEROL (Mg)
Russian, *Wish-Bone Lite* (Lipton)	1 Tbsp	25	none
Russian (Weight Watchers)	1 Tbsp	50	5
Russian, Reduced Calorie (Kraft)	1 Tbsp	30	none
Sesame seed (Generic)	1 Tbsp	68	none
Sour cream & Bacon, *Wish-Bone* (Lipton)	1 Tbsp	70	none
Tartar Sauce, Reduced Calorie (Weight Watchers)	1 Tbsp	35	5
Thousand Island (Kraft)	1 Tbsp	60	5
Thousand Island, *Wish-Bone* (Lipton)	1 Tbsp	70	5
Thousand Island, *Wish-Bone Lite* (Lipton)	1 Tbsp	40	10
Thousand Island (Weight Watchers)	1 Tbsp	50	5
Thousand Island, Reduced Calorie (Kraft)	1 Tbsp	30	5
Thousand Island, Southern Recipe, *Wish-Bone* (Lipton)	1 Tbsp	70	10
Thousand Island & Bacon (Kraft)	1 Tbsp	60	none
Thousand Island w/Bacon, Southern Recipe, *Wish-Bone* (Lipton)	1 Tbsp	60	5

SALT/SALT SUBSTITUTE

Food	Portion	Calories	Cholesterol
Salt, iodized	1 tsp	0	none
Salt Substitute (Diamond)	1 tsp	2	none

SALAMI
(*see* LUNCHEON MEATS/COLD CUTS, TURKEY)

FOOD	PORTION SIZE	CALORIES	CHOLESTEROL (Mg)

SAUCES & SEASONINGS
(*see also* DIPS; GRAVY; NOODLES & PASTA; SALAD DRESSINGS; SOUPS, DRY)

FOOD	PORTION SIZE	CALORIES	CHOLESTEROL (Mg)
Barbecue (Generic)	1 Tbsp	12	none
Bearnaise dry; as prep w/whole milk & butter (Generic)	1 cup	712	189
Bearnaise, dry (Generic)	⅞ oz pkg	90	tr
Catsup	1 Tbsp	16	none
Cheese, dry (Generic)	1¼ oz pkg	158	18
Cheese, dry; as prep w/whole milk (Generic)	2 Tbsp	38	7
Chile (Generic)	1 Tbsp	16	none
Clam (Home recipe)	½ cup	274	87
Cocktail Sauce, *Sauceworks* (Kraft)	1 Tbsp	12	none
Curry, dry (Generic)	1¼ oz pkg	151	tr
Curry, dry; as prep w/whole milk (Generic)	2 Tbsp	34	4
Custard (Home recipe)	2 Tbsp	49	66
Grape (Home recipe)	1 Tbsp	26	none
Hard (Home recipe)	2 Tbsp	142	15
Hollandaise (Home recipe)	2 Tbsp	134	148
Hollandaise, dry butterfat (Generic)	1⅕ oz pkg	187	53
Hollandaise, dry vegetable oil; as prep w/whole milk & butter (Generic)	2 Tbsp	88	24
Hollandaise, *Jiffy* (Home recipe)	2 Tbsp	130	16
Horseradish Sauce (Kraft)	1 Tbsp	50	5
Horseradish, Mustard (Kraft)	1 tsp	4	none
Horseradish, Prepared (Kraft)	1 tsp	4	none
Horseradish, Prepared, Cream Style (Kraft)	1 Tbsp	8	none

FOOD	PORTION SIZE	CALORIES	CHOLESTEROL (Mg)
Italian Paste (Contadina)	2 oz	70	<1
Lemon (Home recipe)	2 Tbsp	57	48
Mushroom, dry (Generic)	1 oz pkg	99	none
Mushroom, dry; as prep w/ whole milk (Generic)	2 Tbsp	28	4
Mustard, Hot, *Sauceworks* (Kraft)	1 Tbsp	35	5
Mustard, Prepared, Pure (Kraft)	1 tsp	4	none
Sour cream, dry (Generic)	1¼ oz pkg	180	28
Sour cream, dry; as prep w/ whole milk (Generic)	2 Tbsp	64	11
Soy sauce (Generic)	1 Tbsp	11	none
Spaghetti, dry (Generic)	¼ pkg (10 g)	28	none
Spaghetti Sauce, *Prego* (Campbell)	½ cup	140	none
Spaghetti Sauce, Extra Thick & Zesty, Flavored w/Meat, *Ragu* (Cheesebrough-Ponds, Inc)	½ cup	100	2
Spaghetti Sauce, Extra Thick & Zesty Plain, *Ragu* (Cheesebrough-Ponds, Inc)	½ cup	100	none
Spaghetti Sauce, Flavored w/ Meat, *Ragu* (Cheesebrough-Ponds, Inc)	½ cup	80	2
Spaghetti Sauce, Home Style w/Mushrooms, *Ragu* (Cheesebrough-Ponds, Inc)	½ cup	70	none
Spaghetti Sauce, Plain, *Ragu* (Cheesebrough-Ponds, Inc)	½ cup	80	none
Spaghetti sauce, w/ mushrooms, dry (Generic)	¼ pkg (10 g)	30	3

FOOD	PORTION SIZE	CALORIES	CHOLESTEROL (Mg)
Spaghetti Sauce, w/ mushrooms, *Prego* (Campbell)	½ cup	140	none
Spaghetti Sauce w/Sweet Peppers & Italian Sausage, *Aunt Millie's* (Prince)	½ cup	64	tr
Steak Sauce, *A-1* (Heublein)	1 Tbsp	14	none
Stroganoff, dry (Generic)	1⅗ oz pkg	161	11
Stroganoff, dry; as prep w/ whole milk & water (Generic)	1 cup	272	38
Sweet & Sour, dry (Generic)	2 oz pkg	221	none
Sweet 'N Sour, Sauceworks (Kraft)	1 Tbsp	20	none
Sweet'n Sour Sauce (Contadina)	½ cup	150	none
Tabasco (McIlhenny)	1 Tbsp	1	none
Tartar (Generic)	1 Tbsp	74	none
Tartar Sauce, *Sauceworks* (Kraft)	1 Tbsp	70	5
Tartar, Hellmann's (CPC International, Inc)	1 Tbsp	71	5
Tartar, low calorie (Generic)	1 Tbsp	31	none
Teriyaki (Generic)	1 Tbsp	15	none
Teriyaki, dry (Generic)	1⅗ oz pkg	130	none
Tomato (Contadina)	½ cup	45	none
Tomato Paste (Contadina)	2 oz	50	none
Tomato, Italian style (Contadina)	½ cup	40	none
Western BBQ, *Sauceworks* (Kraft)	2 Tbsp	50	none
White, dry (Generic)	1¾ oz pkg	230	none
White, dry; as prep w/whole milk (Generic)	1 cup	241	34

FOOD	PORTION SIZE	CALORIES	CHOLESTEROL (Mg)
Worchestershire (Lea & Perrins)	1 Tbsp	59	none

SAUSAGE

(*see also* FRANKFURTER, HAM, LUNCHEON MEATS/COLD CUTS, MEAT SUBSTITUTES, TURKEY)

Sources for the following sausage values did not always indicate whether or not a product is cooked. When the information was given, it is noted. In all other cases, it should be assumed that values given are for the uncooked product, or a cured ready-to-eat product.

FOOD	PORTION SIZE	CALORIES	CHOLESTEROL (Mg)
Bratwurst, Fully Cooked (Hillshire Farm)	3½ oz	305	28
Braunschweiger, Liver Sausage (Oscar Mayer)	1 oz	96	41
Breakfast Links, Beef, *Brown 'N Serve;* cooked (Swift)	1 link (2 oz)	113	17
Breakfast Links, Lights; cooked (Jones)	3½ oz	240	73
Breakfast Links, Pork, *Brown 'N Serve Original;* cooked (Swift)	1 link (2 oz)	130	20
Breakfast, Little Friers, Pork (Oscar Mayer)	1 link (20 g)	77	16
Breakfast Little Sausage; cooked (Jones)	1 link (2 oz)	221	38
Breakfast Sausage, Turkey (Louis Rich)	1 oz	59	23
Breakfast, Sausage, Pork (Jimmy Dean)	1 link (2 oz)	200	58
Cheddarwurst (Hillshire Farm)	3½ oz	343	30
Italian Sausage, Hot, before cooking (Hillshire Farm)	3½ oz	317	37

FOOD	PORTION SIZE	CALORIES	CHOLESTEROL (Mg)
Italian Sausage, Mild, before cooking (Hillshire Farm)	3½ oz	317	26
Knockwurst (Hillshire Farm)	3½ oz	324	43
Mettwurst (Hillshire Farm)	3½ oz	337	26
Mettwurst, Hot, Smoked (Kahn's)	3½ oz	320	55
Polska Kielbasa (Kahn's)	3½ oz	324	57
Polska Kielbasa, Beef (Hillshire Farm)	3½ oz	334	29
Polska Kielbasa, Endless (Hillshire Farm)	3½ oz	336	23
Pork, cooked (Generic)	½ cup	333	62
Smoked link, pork (Generic)	1 link (16 g)	62	11
Smoked link, pork & beef (Generic)	1 link (16 g)	54	11
Smoked link, pork, beef, flour & nonfat milk added (Generic)	1 link (16 g)	54	11
Smoked Links (Hillshire Farm)	3½ oz	337	20
Smoked links, country style (Generic)	1	148	38
Smoked, Beef (Hillshire Farm)	3½ oz	331	29
Smoked, Endless (Hillshire Farm)	3½ oz	334	20
Smoked, Turkey (Louis Rich)	1 oz	55	20
Smokie Links (Oscar Mayer)	1 link (43 g)	124	27
Smokies, Beef (Oscar Mayer)	1 link (43 g)	122	27
Smokies, Cheese (Oscar Mayer)	1 link (43 g)	127	28
Smokies, Little (Oscar Mayer)	1 link (9 g)	28	6

FOOD	PORTION SIZE	CALORIES	CHOLESTEROL (Mg)
Summer Sausage, Turkey (Louis Rich)	1 oz	52	23
Summer, Sausage, Thuringer Cervelat (Oscar Mayer)	1 slice (23 g)	73	17
Summer sausage, thuringer cervelat, beef, pork (Generic)	1 slice (23 g)	80	16
Vienna canned, beef & pork (Generic)	1 sausage (16 g)	45	8

SCONES
(*see* BREAD & ROLLS)

SEASONINGS
(*see* SAUCES)

SHAKE 'N BAKE
(*see* CHICKEN)

SODA
(*see also* MINERAL WATER)

Cherry Coke (Generic)	12 oz	154	none
Club soda (Generic)	8 oz	0	none
Coca Cola Classic	12 oz	144	none
Coca Cola	12 oz	154	none
Cola (Generic)	8 oz	104	none

FOOD	PORTION SIZE	CALORIES	CHOLESTEROL (Mg)
Cola, low-calorie (Generic)	8 oz	2	none
Cream Soda (Generic)	8 oz	128	none
Diet Coke	12 oz	.9	none
Diet Sprite	12 oz	3	none
Dr Pepper	12 oz	144	none
Dr Pepper, Sugar-Free	12 oz	3	none
Fanta Ginger Ale	12 oz	126	none
Fanta Grape	12 oz	168	none
Fanta Orange	12 oz	164	none
Fanta Root Beer	12 oz	158	none
Fresca	12 oz	4	none
Ginger ale (Generic)	8 oz	80	none
Grape drink, canned (Generic)	8 oz	112	none
Grape soda (Generic)	8 oz	104	none
Lemon/lime soda (Generic)	8 oz	96	none
Mellow Yello	12 oz	172	none
Mr. Pibb	12 oz	142	none
Orange soda (Generic)	8 oz	120	none
Quinine water	12 oz	113	none
Ramblin' Root Beer	12 oz	158	none
Root Beer (Generic)	8 oz	104	none
7-up	12 oz	155	none
7-up diet	12 oz	4	none
Seltzer (Generic)	8 oz	0	none
Sprite	12 oz	142	none
Tab	12 oz	1	none
Tonic (Generic)	8 oz	80	none

SOUFFLE

FOOD	PORTION SIZE	CALORIES	CHOLESTEROL (Mg)
Cheese (Home recipe)	1 cup	308	196
Pineapple (Home recipe)	1 cup	244	141

FOOD	PORTION SIZE	CALORIES	CHOLESTEROL (Mg)

SOUPS, CANNED
(*see also* SOUPS, DRY; SOUPS, HOMEMADE)

FOOD	PORTION SIZE	CALORIES	CHOLESTEROL (Mg)
Barley w/beef; as prep w/water (Generic)	1 cup	86	tr
Bean w/bacon; as prep w/water (Generic)	1 cup	172	3
Bean w/frankfurter; as prep w/ water (Generic)	1 cup	188	13
Bean w/ham, chunky, ready-to-serve (Generic)	1 cup	231	22
Beef broth or bouillon, ready-to-serve (Generic)	1 cup	17	tr
Beef, chunky, ready-to-serve (Generic)	1 cup	170	14
Beef noodle; as prep w/water (Generic)	1 cup	83	5
Black bean; as prep w/water (Generic)	1 cup	116	none
Borscht, Low Calorie, ready-to-serve (Manischewitz)	8 oz	20	none
Borscht, With Beets, ready-to-serve (Manischewitz)	8 oz	80	none
Cheese; as prep w/water (Generic)	1 cup	156	30
Cheese; as prep w/whole milk (Generic)	1 cup	231	48
Chicken broth; as prep w/water (Generic)	1 cup	39	none
Chicken gumbo; as prep w/ water (Generic)	1 cup	137	5
Chicken noodle; as prep w/ water (Generic)	1 cup	75	7
Chicken noodle w/meatballs, ready-to-serve (Generic)	1 cup	99	10

FOOD	PORTION SIZE	CALORIES	CHOLESTEROL (Mg)
Chicken, chunky, ready-to-serve (Generic)	1 cup	178	30
Chicken rice; as prep w/water (Generic)	1 cup	60	7
Chicken rice, chunky, ready-to-serve (Generic)	1 cup	127	12
Chicken vegetable; as prep w/water (Generic)	1 cup	75	10
Chicken vegetable, chunky, ready-to-serve (Generic)	1 cup	166	17
Chicken w/dumplings; as prep w/water (Generic)	1 cup	96	34
Chili beef; as prep w/water (Generic)	1 cup	170	13
Clam chowder, Manhattan; as prep w/water (Generic)	1 cup	78	2
Clam chowder, Manhattan, chunky, ready-to-serve (Generic)	1 cup	134	14
Clam chowder, New England; as prep w/water (Generic)	1 cup	95	5
Clam chowder, New England; as prep w/whole milk (Generic)	1 cup	164	22
Clam Chowder, New England; as prep w/whole milk (Doxsee)	6 oz	90	<10
Consomme w/gelatin; as prep w/water (Generic)	1 cup	29	none
Crab, ready-to-serve (Generic)	1 cup	76	10
Cream of asparagus; as prep w/whole milk (Generic)	1 cup	161	22
Cream of celery; as prep w/water (Generic)	1 cup	90	15

FOOD	PORTION SIZE	CALORIES	CHOLESTEROL (Mg)
Cream of celery; as prep w/ whole milk (Generic)	1 cup	164	32
Cream of chicken; as prep w/ water (Generic)	1 cup	117	10
Cream of mushroom; as prep w/whole milk (Generic)	1 cup	203	20
Cream of chicken; ready-to-serve (Generic)	1 cup	191	27
Cream of mushroom; as prep w/water (Generic)	1 cup	129	2
Cream of potato; as prep w/ water (Generic)	1 cup	73	5
Cream of potato; as prep w/ whole milk (Generic)	1 cup	149	22
Cream of shrimp; as prep w/ water (Generic)	1 cup	90	17
Cream of shrimp; as prep w/ whole milk (Generic)	1 cup	164	35
Escarole, ready-to-serve (Generic)	1 cup	27	2
Gazpacho, ready-to-serve (Generic)	1 cup	56	none
Green pea; as prep w/water (Generic)	1 cup	165	none
Green pea; as prep w/whole milk (Generic)	1 cup	239	18
Lentil w/ham; ready-to-serve (Generic)	1 cup	139	7
Minestrone; as prep w/water (Generic)	1 cup	82	2
Minestrone, chunky, ready-to-serve (Generic)	1 cup	127	5
Mushroom w/beef stock; as prep w/water (Generic)	1 cup	85	7

FOOD	PORTION SIZE	CALORIES	CHOLESTEROL (Mg)
Mushroom w/beef stock; as prep w/whole milk (Generic)	1 cup	207	18
Onion; as prep w/water (Generic)	1 cup	58	none
Oyster stew; as prep w/water (Generic)	1 cup	58	14
Oyster stew; as prep w/whole milk (Generic)	1 cup	135	32
Pepper pot; as prep w/water (Generic)	1 cup	241	10
Scotch broth; as prep w/water (Generic)	1 cup	80	5
Split pea w/ham; as prep w/water (Generic)	1 cup	190	8
Split pea w/ham, chunky, ready-to-serve (Generic)	1 cup	185	7
Stockpot; as prep w/water (Generic)	1 cup	99	5
Tomato; as prep w/water (Generic)	1 cup	86	none
Tomato; as prep w/whole milk (Generic)	1 cup	160	17
Tomato beef w/noodle; as prep w/water (Generic)	1 cup	139	5
Tomato bisque; as prep w/water (Generic)	1 cup	123	5
Tomato bisque; as prep w/ whole milk (Generic)	1 cup	198	23
Turkey, chunky; as prep w/ water (Generic)	1 cup	135	9
Tomato rice; as prep w/water (Generic)	1 cup	119	2
Turkey noodle; as prep w/water (Generic)	1 cup	68	5

FOOD	PORTION SIZE	CALORIES	CHOLESTEROL (Mg)
Turkey vegetable; as prep w/ water (Generic)	1 cup	72	2
Vegetable w/beef; as prep w/ water (Generic)	1 cup	78	5
Vegetable w/beef broth; as prep w/water (Generic)	1 cup	82	2
Vegetable, chunky, ready-to-serve (Generic)	1 cup	122	none
Vegetarian vegetable; as prep w/water (Generic)	1 cup	72	none

SOUPS, DRY
(*see also* DIPS; GRAVY; SALAD DRESSINGS; SAUCES; SOUPS, CANNED; SOUPS, HOMEMADE)

FOOD	PORTION SIZE	CALORIES	CHOLESTEROL (Mg)
Bean w/bacon; as prep w/water (Generic)	1 cup	106	3
Beef broth or bouillon, dry (Generic)	1/5 oz pkg	14	1
Beef broth or bouillon; as prep w/water (Generic)	1 cup	20	none
Beef broth, dry (Generic)	1 cube	6	tr
Beef Flavor Noodle, *Cup-a-Soup;* as prep w/water (Lipton)	6 oz	45	15
Beef noodle, dry (Generic)	1/3 pkg	30	1
Beef noodle; as prep w/water (Generic)	1 cup	40	3
Beef, *Cup-a-Soup, Trim;* as prep w/water (Lipton)	6 oz	10	none
Beefy Tomato, *Cup-a-Soup, Trim;* as prep w/water (Lipton)	6 oz	10	none

FOOD	PORTION SIZE	CALORIES	CHOLESTEROL (Mg)
Cauliflower; as prep w/water (Generic)	1 cup	69	tr
Chicken broth or bouillon; as prep w/water (Generic)	1 cup	22	tr
Chicken flavor, *Cup-a-Soup;* as prep w/water (Lipton)	6 oz	25	5
Chicken Flavored, *Lots-a-Noodles;* as prep w/water (Lipton)	7 oz	120	30
Chicken Noodle, *Cup-a-Soup;* as prep w/water (Lipton)	6 oz	90	15
Chicken noodle; as prep w/water (Generic)	1 cup	53	3
Chicken rice; as prep w/water (Generic)	1 cup	61	3
Chicken Vegetable, *Cup-a-Soup;* as prep w/water (Lipton)	1 cup	40	5
Chicken vegetable; as prep w/water (Generic)	1 cup	50	3
Chicken w/Rice, *Cup-a-Soup;* as prep w/water (Lipton)	6 oz	45	5
Chicken, *Cup-a-Soup, Trim;* as prep w/water (Lipton)	6 oz	10	none
Consomme w/gelatin; as prep w/water (Generic)	1 cup	17	none
Cream of asparagus; as prep w/water (Generic)	1 cup	58	tr
Cream of celery; prep w/water (Generic)	1 cup	63	tr
Cream Of Chicken, *Cup-a-Soup;* as prep w/water (Lipton)	6 oz	80	none

FOOD	PORTION SIZE	CALORIES	CHOLESTEROL (Mg)
Cream of chicken, dry (Generic)	⅔ pkg	80	2
Cream Of Chicken, *Lots-a-Noodles;* as prep w/water (Lipton)	7 oz	150	35
Cream Of Mushroom, *Cup-a-Soup;* as prep w/water (Lipton)	6 oz	80	none
Cream of vegetable, dry (Generic)	⅗ oz	79	tr
French Onion, *Cup-a-Soup, Trim;* as prep w/water (Lipton)	6 oz	10	none
Garden Vegetable, *Lots-a-Noodles;* as prep w/water (Lipton)	7 oz	130	30
Green Pea, *Cup-a-Soup;* as prep w/water (Lipton)	6 oz	120	none
Herb Chicken, *Cup-a-Soup, Trim;* as prep w/water (Lipton)	6 oz	10	none
Herb Vegetable, *Cup-a-Soup;* as prep w/water (Lipton)	6 oz	10	none
Leek, dry (Generic)	2¾ oz pkg	294	9
Minestrone Mix; as prep w/water (Manischewitz)	6 oz	50	none
Minestrone, dry (Generic)	2¾ oz pkg	279	6
Mushroom, dry (Generic)	⅗ oz pkg	74	tr
Onion, *Cup-a-Soup;* as prep w/water (Lipton)	6 oz	30	none
Onion, dry (Generic)	¼ oz	21	tr
Split Pea Mix; as prep w/water (Manischewitz)	6 oz	45	none
Split pea, dry (Generic)	1 oz pkg	77	tr

FOOD	PORTION SIZE	CALORIES	CHOLESTEROL (Mg)
Spring Vegetable, *Cup-a-Soup;* as prep w/water (Lipton)	6 oz	40	5
Tomato vegetable, dry (Generic)	1⅓ oz	125	1
Tomato, *Cup-a-Soup;* as prep w/water (Lipton)	6 oz	80	none
Tomato, dry (Generic)	¾ oz	77	1
Vegetable beef, dry (Generic)	2⅖ oz	256	6
Vegetable Mix; as prep w/water (Manischewitz)	6 oz	50	none

SOUPS, HOMEMADE
(*see also* SOUPS, CANNED; SOUPS, DRY)

FOOD	PORTION SIZE	CALORIES	CHOLESTEROL (Mg)
Corn chowder (Home recipe)	1 cup	233	75
Greek (Home recipe)	¾ cup	63	83
Lentil (Home recipe)	1 cup	175	none
Mock turtle (Home recipe)	1 cup	256	164
Potato (Home recipe)	1 cup	201	37
Seafood chowder (Home recipe)	1 cup	170	68
Vegetable (Home recipe)	1 cup	70	none
Vegetable beef (Home recipe)	1 cup	320	54
Wonton (Home recipe)	1 cup	205	89

SOUR CREAM
(*see also* CREAM, WHIPPED TOPPING)

FOOD	PORTION SIZE	CALORIES	CHOLESTEROL (Mg)
Sour Cream (Land O Lakes)	1 Tbsp	25	5
Sour Cream (Generic)	1 Tbsp	31	7
Imitation, non-dairy, cultured (Generic)	1 Tbsp	30	none

FOOD	PORTION SIZE	CALORIES	CHOLESTEROL (Mg)
Imitation Sour Cream (Pet)	1 Tbsp	25	none
Low Fat, *Lite Delite* (Friendship)	2 Tbsp (1 oz)	35	8
Low Fat, *Lean Cream* (Land O Lakes)	1 Tbsp	20	4
Low Fat, *Lean Cream* w/Chives (Land O Lakes)	1 Tbsp	20	4

SOY
(*see also* BEANS)

FOOD	PORTION SIZE	CALORIES	CHOLESTEROL (Mg)
Flour, defatted (Generic)	3.5 oz	326	none
Milk (Generic)	1 cup	87	none
Miso	1 Tbsp	36	none
Natto	1 Tbsp	23	none
Soy Sauce, shoyu (Generic)	1 Tbsp	9	none
Soy Sauce, Tamari (Generic)	1 Tbsp	11	none
Soybeans; boiled	½ cup	149	none
Soybeans; dry roasted	½ cup	387	none
Soybeans; roasted	½ cup	405	none
Tempeh	1 Tbsp	21	none
Tofu, cheese	3½ oz	72	none

SPAGHETTI
(*see* NOODLES & PASTA)

SPAGHETTI SAUCE
(*see* SAUCES)

FOOD	PORTION SIZE	CALORIES	CHOLESTEROL (Mg)

SPARE RIBS
(*see* PORK)

STEW

FOOD	PORTION SIZE	CALORIES	CHOLESTEROL (Mg)
Beef w/vegetables (Home recipe)	1 cup	209	61
Beef w/vegetables, canned (Generic)	1 cup	186	33
Crab (Home recipe)	1 cup	208	73
Frankfurter (Home recipe)	¾ cup	291	42
Lamb (Home recipe)	¾ cup	124	29
Oyster (Home recipe)	1 cup	278	100
Shrimp (Home recipe)	1 cup	207	79
Turkey (Home recipe)	1 cup	336	138

SQUAB

FOOD	PORTION SIZE	CALORIES	CHOLESTEROL (Mg)
Squab (Pigeon), breast w/o skin	3½ oz	135	91

STUFFING/DRESSING

FOOD	PORTION SIZE	CALORIES	CHOLESTEROL (Mg)
Beef; as prep w/butter (Stove Top)	½ cup	180	20
Bread w/eggs (Home recipe)	½ cup	107	75
Bread, *Americana New England;* as prep w/butter (Stove Top)	½ cup	180	20
Bread, *Americana San Francisco;* as prep w/butter (Stove Top)	½ cup	170	20

FOOD	PORTION SIZE	CALORIES	CHOLESTEROL (Mg)
Bread, Cube Stuffing; as prep w/butter (Pepperidge Farm)	1 oz	110	16
Bread, Cubed Country Style; as prep w/butter (Pepperidge Farm)	1 oz	110	16
Chicken flavor; as prep w/butter (Stove Top)	½ cup	180	20
Chicken Flavor Stuffing Mix, *Flexible Serving;* as prep w/ butter (Stove Top)	½ cup	170	15
Corn Bread; as prep w/butter (Stove Top)	½ cup	170	20
Corn Bread Stuffing Mix, *Flexible Serving;* as prep w/ butter (Stove Top)	½ cup	170	15
Corn Stuffing; as prep w/butter (Pepperidge Farm)	1 oz	110	16
Herb, Homestyle Stuffing Mix, *Flexible Serving;* as prep w/ butter (Stove Top)	½ cup	170	15
Herb Seasoned Stuffing; as prep w/butter (Pepperidge Farm)	1 oz	110	16
Herbs, Savory; as prep w/ butter (Stove Top)	½ cup	180	20
Pork; as prep w/butter (Stove Top)	½ cup	170	20
Rice, Long Grain & Wild; as prep w/butter (Stove Top)	½ cup	180	20
Rice, Wild; as prep w/butter (Stove Top)	½ cup	180	20
Sausage (Home recipe)	½ cup	292	12
Turkey; as prep w/butter (Stove Top)	½ cup	170	20

FOOD	PORTION SIZE	CALORIES	CHOLESTEROL (Mg)

SUGAR/SUGAR SUBSTITUTES

FOOD	PORTION SIZE	CALORIES	CHOLESTEROL (Mg)
Equal	1 pkg	4	none
Brown	1 Tbsp	52	none
White	1 tsp	16	none
Sweet 'n Low	1 pkg	4	none

SUNDAE TOPPINGS

FOOD	PORTION SIZE	CALORIES	CHOLESTEROL (Mg)
Butterscotch, artificially flavored (Kraft)	1 Tbsp	60	none
Caramel (Kraft)	1 Tbsp	60	none
Cherry (Smucker's)	1 Tbsp	53	none
Chocolate Flavored Syrup (Hershey)	3½ oz	260	none
Hot Fudge (Kraft)	1 Tbsp	70	none
Marshmallow (Smucker's)	1 Tbsp	68	none
Walnut (Kraft)	1 Tbsp	90	none

SWEETBREADS

FOOD	PORTION SIZE	CALORIES	CHOLESTEROL (Mg)
Beef; cooked	3 oz	244	780
Calve's; braised	3½ oz	168	466
Lamb; braised	3½ oz	175	466

SYRUP
(*see* MILK FLAVORINGS, SUNDAE TOPPINGS)

FOOD	PORTION SIZE	CALORIES	CHOLESTEROL (Mg)

TACO BELL

FOOD	PORTION SIZE	CALORIES	CHOLESTEROL (Mg)
Bean Burrito	1	360	14
Bean Burrito, Green	1	354	14
Beef Burrito	1	402	59
Beef Burrito, Green	1	396	59
Beefy Tostado	1	313	40
Beefy Tostado, Green	1	316	40
Bell Beefer	1	312	38
Bell Beefer, Green	1	306	39
Burrito Supreme	1	422	35
Burrito Supreme Platter	1	774	79
Burrito Supreme Platter, Green	1	762	79
Burrito Supreme, Green	1	416	35
Cinnamon Crispies	1	266	2
Combo Burrito	1	381	36
Combo Burrito, Green	1	375	36
Double Beef Burrito Supreme	1	465	59
Double Beef Burrito Supreme, Green	1	459	59
Enchirito	1	382	56
Enchirito, Green	1	370	56
Hot Taco Sauce	1 packet	3	none
Nachos	1	356	9
Nachos Bellgrande	1	719	43
Pintos & Cheese	1	194	19
Pintos & Cheese, Green	1	189	19
Pizzazz Pizza	1	714	81
Seafood Salad	1	920	123
Seafood Salad w/o Dressing	1	648	82
Seafood Salad w/o Shell	1	224	78
Soft Taco	1	228	32
Taco	1	184	32
Taco Bellgrande	1	351	55
Taco Bellgrande Platter	1	1002	80

FOOD	PORTION SIZE	CALORIES	CHOLESTEROL (Mg)
Taco *Bellgrande* Platter, Green	1	990	80
Taco Light	1	411	57
Taco Light Platter	1	1062	82
Taco Light Platter, Green	1	1051	82
Taco Salad	1	949	85
Taco Salad w/o Beans	1	821	80
Taco Salad w/o Salsa	1	931	85
Taco Salad w/o Shell	1	523	82
Taco Salad w/Ranch Dressing	1	1204	126
Taco Sauce	1 packet	2	none
Tostado	1	243	18
Tostado, Green	1	238	18

TACOS

FOOD	PORTION SIZE	CALORIES	CHOLESTEROL (Mg)
Taco salad (Home recipe)	1 cup	292	71
Taco Verde Blanco y Rojo (Home recipe)	1	296	38

TALLOW
(*see* FATS)

TAMALE

FOOD	PORTION SIZE	CALORIES	CHOLESTEROL (Mg)
Tamale (Home recipe)	1 avg	155	10

TARTAR SAUCE
(*see* SAUCES & SEASONINGS)

FOOD	PORTION SIZE	CALORIES	CHOLESTEROL (Mg)

TEXTURED VEGETABLE PROTEIN (TVP)

TVP (Generic)	1 oz	80	none

TOFUTTI
(*see* ICE CREAM & FROZEN DESSERTS)

TONGUE

Beef; cooked	3 oz	241	91
Pork; cooked	3 oz	230	124

TORTILLA
(*see also* BREAD & ROLLS)

Tortilla; baked or steamed (Home recipe)	1	43	none
Tortilla casserole (Home recipe)	¾ cup	230	33
Tortilla, Corn *Masa Harina Mix* (Quaker)	1 cup	421	none
Tortilla, Wheat *Masa Tirgo Mix* (Quaker)	1 cup	458	none

TUNA
(*see* FISH)

TUNA HELPER
(*see* NOODLES & PASTA, RICE)

FOOD	PORTION SIZE	CALORIES	CHOLESTEROL (Mg)

TURKEY
(*see also* FRANKFURTER, HAM, LUNCHEON MEATS/COLD CUTS, SAUSAGE, MEAT SUBSTITUTES)

FOOD	PORTION SIZE	CALORIES	CHOLESTEROL (Mg)
Back, w/skin; roasted (Generic)	9 oz	530	281
Back, w/o skin; roasted (Generic)	7 oz	326	182
Bologna, Turkey (Louis Rich)	1 slice (1 oz)	58	19
Breast Fillet w/Cheese (Land O Lakes)	5 oz	300	35
Breast, w/skin, prebasted; cooked (Generic)	3 oz	107	36
Breast, w/skin; roasted (Generic)	12 oz	526	310
Breast, w/o skin; roasted (Generic)	3 oz	115	71
Breast, Barbecued (Louis Rich)	1 oz	38	10
Breast, Hickory Smoked (Louis Rich)	1 oz	35	13
Breast, Oven Cooked, *Bronze Label* (Land O Lakes)	3 oz	100	50
Breast, Oven Cooked, Browned *Gold Label* (Land O Lakes)	3 oz	120	55
Breast, Oven Cooked, *Silver Label* (Land O Lakes)	3 oz	100	50
Breast, Oven Cooked, Skinless, *Gold Label* (Land O Lakes)	3 oz	90	50
Breast, Oven Cooked, Skin On, *Gold Label* (Land O Lakes)	3 oz	120	55
Breast, Oven Roasted (Louis Rich)	1 oz	36	10
Breast, Ready-To-Serve (Louis Rich)	1 oz	51	12

FOOD	PORTION SIZE	CALORIES	CHOLESTEROL (Mg)
Breast, ready-to-serve (Generic)	1 slice (21 g)	23	9
Breast, Smoked (Generic)	1 slice (21 g)	20	7
Breast, Smoked (Louis Rich)	1 slice	21	7
Breast, Smoked, Chunk (Louis Rich)	1 oz	34	11
Breast, Tender Loins; cooked (Louis Rich)	1 oz	41	9
Dark Meat, w/skin; roasted (Generic)	3 oz	155	99
Dark meat, w/o skin; roasted, chopped (Generic)	½ cup	113	78
Drum Sticks (Louis Rich)	1 oz	55	33
Fat (Generic)	1 cup	1846	209
Franks, Turkey (Louis Rich)	1 link (45 g)	103	40
Franks, Turkey, Cheese (Louis Rich)	1 link (45 g)	108	39
Ground Meat; cooked (Louis Rich)	1 oz	61	24
Ham, Turkey (Louis Rich)	1 oz	34	18
Ham, Turkey, Chopped (Louis Rich)	1 oz	42	17
Leg, w/skin; roasted (Generic)	9 oz	416	171
Leg, w/o skin; roasted (Generic)	9 oz	356	267
Light meat, w/skin; roasted (Generic)	3 oz	139	81
Light meat, w/o skin; roasted, chopped (Generic)	½ cup	98	60
Light & dark meat, w/o skin; roasted, chopped (Generic)	½ cup	105	69

FOOD	PORTION SIZE	CALORIES	CHOLESTEROL (Mg)
Loaf (Home recipe)	4″ sq slice	263	138
Luncheon Loaf, Turkey (Louis Rich)	1 oz	43	14
Pastrami, Turkey (Louis Rich)	1 slice (1 oz)	33	17
Patties, Turkey (Land O Lakes)	2¼ oz	170	30
Potpie (Home recipe)	1	710	122
Salami, Cotto, Turkey (Louis Rich)	1 oz	52	22
Salami, Turkey (Louis Rich)	1 slice (1 oz)	52	19
Sausage, Breakfast (Louis Rich)	1 oz	59	23
Sausage, Smoked (Louis Rich)	1 oz	55	19
Sausage, Summer (Louis Rich)	1 oz	52	23
Skin; roasted (Generic)	1 oz	85	41
Smoked, Turkey (Louis Rich)	1 oz	33	12
Sticks, Turkey (Land O Lakes)	2 oz	150	25
Thigh; cooked (Louis Rich)	1 oz	65	28
Turkey roll, light meat (Generic)	1 oz	42	12
Turkey Roll, Light Meat, *Red Label* (Land O Lakes)	3 oz	110	50
Turkey roll, light & dark meat (Generic)	1 oz	24	16
Turkey Roll, Light & Dark Meat, *Red Label* (Land O Lakes)	3 oz	110	50
W/Gravy, Light & Dark Meat (Land O Lakes)	3 oz	120	20
W/Gravy, Light Meat (Land O Lakes)	3 oz	110	20
Whole Turkey, cooked (Louis Rich)	1 oz	57	18
Wing Drumettes, cooked (Louis Rich)	1 oz	53	20

FOOD	PORTION SIZE	CALORIES	CHOLESTEROL (Mg)
Wing w/skin; roasted (Generic)	1 piece (2 oz)	186	103
Wing w/o skin; roasted (Generic)	1 piece (2 oz)	98	61
Wings; cooked (Louis Rich)	1 oz	54	26

VEAL
(*see also* BEEF)

Cutlet, w/o bone, not trimmed; broiled	3 oz	184	86
Loaf (Home recipe)	4.5 oz	270	135
Loin chop, w/bone, fully trimmed	4¾ oz raw	143	68
Loin chop, w/bone, fully trimmed	6½ oz raw	194	93
Loin chop, w/bone, not trimmed	4¾ oz raw	190	82
Loin chop, w/bone, not trimmed	6½ oz raw	257	111
Loin roast, w/o bone, fully trimmed; roasted	3 oz	130	84
Loin roast, w/o bone, not trimmed; roasted	3 oz	199	86
Parmigiana (Home recipe)	4 oz	279	136
Rib chop, w/bone, not trimmed; cooked	3.5 oz	269	99
Round, not trimmed; cooked, chopped	½ cup	151	71
Round, not trimmed; cooked, ground	½ cup	119	56
Round, patty; cooked	3″ diam (3 oz)	184	86

FOOD	PORTION SIZE	CALORIES	CHOLESTEROL (Mg)
Shoulder roast, w/o bone, fully trimmed; braised	3 oz	170	84
Shoulder roast, w/o bone, not trimmed; braised	3 oz	200	86
Shoulder steak, w/bone, fully trimmed; cooked	8 oz raw	196	97

VEGETABLES
(*see also* BEANS, POTATOES)

FOOD	PORTION SIZE	CALORIES	CHOLESTEROL (Mg)
Alfalfa sprouts	1 Tbsp	1	none
Amaranth	1 leaf	4	none
Artichoke; cooked	1 med	53	none
Artichoke Hearts, *Deluxe*, frzn (Birds Eye)	3 oz	30	none
Asparagus; cooked	4 spears	15	none
Asparagus Cuts, frzn (Birds Eye)	3.3 oz	25	none
Asparagus Spears, frzn (Birds Eye)	3.3 oz	25	none
Bamboo shoot; cooked	1	18	none
Beets; cooked	½ cup	26	none
Beets, Harvard; cooked (Home recipe)	½ cup	89	none
Beets, pickled	½ cup	75	none
Broccoli w/Cheese Sauce, frzn (Birds Eye)	5 oz	120	5
Broccoli, Baby Carrots & Water Chestnuts, frzn (Birds Eye)	3.3 oz	35	none
Broccoli, Baby Spears, *Deluxe*, frzn (Birds Eye)	3.3 oz	30	none
Broccoli, Carrots & Pasta Twists, frzn (Birds Eye)	3.3 oz	90	none

FOOD	PORTION SIZE	CALORIES	CHOLESTEROL (Mg)
Broccoli, Cauliflower & Carrots w/Cheese Sauce, frzn (Birds Eye)	5 oz	100	5
Broccoli, Cauliflower & Carrots, frzn (Birds Eye)	3.2 oz	25	none
Broccoli & Cauliflower w/ Creamy Italian Cheese Sauce, frzn (Birds Eye)	4.5 oz	90	none
Broccoli, Chopped, frzn (Birds Eye)	3.3 oz	25	none
Broccoli, Corn, & Red Peppers, frzn (Birds Eye)	3.2 oz	50	none
Broccoli, Cuts, frzn (Birds Eye)	3.3 oz (1 stalk)	25	none
Broccoli, Florets, *Deluxe*, frzn (Birds Eye)	3.3 oz	25	none
Broccoli, Green Beans, Pearl Onions & Red Peppers, frzn (Birds Eye)	3.2 oz	25	none
Broccoli, raw	1 stalk	32	none
Broccoli, Red Peppers, Bamboo Shoots, Mushrooms, frzn (Birds Eye)	3.2 oz	25	none
Broccoli, Spear, frzn (Birds Eye)	3.3 oz	25	none
Broccoli, w/Creamy Italian Cheese Sauce, frzn (Birds Eye)	4.5 oz	90	15
Broccoli & Cauliflower w/ Creamy Italian Cheese Sauce, frzn (Birds Eye)	4.5 oz	90	none
Brussels Sprouts, frzn (Birds Eye)	3.3 oz	35	none

FOOD	PORTION SIZE	CALORIES	CHOLESTEROL (Mg)
Brussels Sprouts, Baby, w/ Cheese Sauce, frzn (Birds Eye)	4½ oz	110	5
Brussels Sprouts, Cauliflower & Carrots, frzn (Birds Eye)	3.2 oz	30	none
Cabbage; cooked	½ cup	16	none
Cabbage, raw	½ cup	8	none
Cabbage, red, raw	½ cup	10	none
Carrot juice	½ cup	49	none
Carrot, canned (Generic)	⅔ cup	31	none
Carrot; cooked	1 med	31	none
Carrot raisin salad (Home recipe)	½ cup	153	none
Carrot, Whole Baby, *Deluxe*, frzn (Birds Eye)	3.3 oz	4	none
Carrots, Baby Peas & Pearl Onions, *Deluxe,* frzn (Birds Eye)	3.3 oz	50	none
Cauliflower, frzn (Birds Eye)	3.3 oz	25	none
Cauliflower, Baby Whole Carrots & Snow Pea Pods, frzn (Birds Eye)	3.2 oz	30	none
Cauliflower w/Cheese Sauce, frzn (Birds Eye)	5 oz	110	5
Celery, raw	1 stalk	6	none
Chayote, raw	1 cup	32	none
Chicory greens, raw	½ cup	21	none
Chinese cabbage; cooked	½ cup	10	none
Chives, raw; chopped	1 tsp	0	none
Collards; cooked	½ cup	21	none
Corn, canned (Generic)	½ cup	66	none
Corn, canned, cream style (Generic)	½ cup	93	none

FOOD	PORTION SIZE	CALORIES	CHOLESTEROL (Mg)
Corn, Green Beans & Pasta Curls, frzn (Birds Eye)	3.3 oz	110	none
Corn kernels, frzn (Generic)	½ cup	67	none
Corn On The Cob, frzn (Birds Eye)	4″ ear	120	none
Corn pudding (Home recipe)	⅔ cup	181	153
Corn, Tender Sweet, *Deluxe*, frzn (Birds Eye)	3.3 oz	80	none
Cucumber, raw	½ cup	7	none
Green beans, frzn (Generic)	½ cup	26	none
Green Beans, Cut, frzn (Birds Eye)	3 oz	25	none
Green Beans, French Cut, frzn (Birds Eye)	3 oz	25	none
Green beans, French style, canned (Generic)	3½ oz	15	none
Green beans, French style, frzn (Generic)	⅖ cup	26	none
Green Beans, French w/Toasted Almonds, frzn (Birds Eye)	3.3 oz	50	none
Green beans, Italian, canned (Generic)	⅔ cup	22	none
Green beans, Italian, frozen (Generic)	⅔ cup	37	none
Green Beans, Italian, frzn (Birds Eye)	3 oz	30	none
Green Beans, Whole, *Deluxe*, frzn (Birds Eye)	3 oz	30	none
Green Beans & Spaetzle, Bavarian Style Recipe, *International*, frzn (Birds Eye)	3.3 oz	110	10
Lima beans; cooked	½ cup	104	none
Lima Beans, Baby, frzn (Birds Eye)	3.3 oz	130	none

FOOD	PORTION SIZE	CALORIES	CHOLESTEROL (Mg)
Lima Beans, Fordhook, frzn (Birds Eye)	3.3 oz	100	none
Mixed vegetables, canned (Generic)	⅗ cup	22	none
Mixed Vegetables, frzn (Birds Eye)	3.3 oz	60	none
Mixed Vegetables, Chinese Style, *International*, frzn (Birds Eye)	3.3 oz	80	none
Mixed Vegetables, Chinese Style, *International Stir-Fry*, frzn (Birds Eye)	3.3 oz	35	none
Mixed Vegetables, Chow Mein Style, *International*, frzn (Birds Eye)	3.3 oz	90	none
Mixed Vegetables, Italian Style, *International*, frzn (Birds Eye)	3.3 oz	110	none
Mixed Vegetables, Japanese Style, *International*, frzn (Birds Eye)	3.3 oz	100	none
Mixed Vegetables, Japanese Style, *International Stir-Fry*, frzn (Birds Eye)	3.3 oz	30	none
Mixed Vegetables, Mandarin Style, *International*, frzn (Birds Eye)	3.3 oz	90	none
Mixed Vegetables, New England Style, *International*, frzn (Birds eye)	3.3 oz	130	none
Mixed Vegetables, San Francisco Style, *International*, frzn (Birds Eye)	3.3 oz	100	none

FOOD	PORTION SIZE	CALORIES	CHOLESTEROL (Mg)
Mixed Vegetables, w/Onion Sauce (Birds Eye)	2.6 oz	100	none
Mung bean sprouts	½ cup	113	none
Navy bean sprouts	½ cup	35	none
Onion, chopped, frzn (Generic)	¼ cup	8	none
Onion, raw, sliced	1 cup	40	none
Onions, Small, Whole, frzn (Birds Eye)	4 oz	40	none
Onions, Small, w/Cream Sauce, frzn (Birds Eye)	3.3 oz	110	none
Pasta Primavera Style, *International*, frzn (Birds Eye)	3.3 oz	120	5
Peas, cooked	⅔ cup	71	none
Peas & Pearl Onions w/Cheese, frzn (Birds Eye)	5 oz	140	5
Peas & Pearl Onions, frzn (Birds Eye)	3.3 oz	70	none
Peas, Green, frzn (Birds Eye)	3.3 oz	80	none
Peas, Green & Potatoes, w/ Cream Sauce, frzn (Birds Eye)	2.6 oz	130	none
Peas, Green & Rice w/ Mushrooms, frzn (Birds Eye)	2.3 oz	110	none
Peas, raw	¾ cup	84	none
Peas, Green, Shells & Mushrooms w/Cream Sauce (Birds Eye)	½ cup	129	tr
Peas, Tender Tiny, *Deluxe,* frzn (Birds Eye)	3.3 oz	60	none
Peas, Green, w/Cream Sauce (Birds Eye)	2.6 oz	120	none
Pinto beans	3⅓ oz	152	none
Shellie beans, canned (Generic)	½ cup	37	none
Snap beans, canned (Generic)	½ cup	17	none

FOOD	PORTION SIZE	CALORIES	CHOLESTEROL (Mg)
Spinach, Chopped, frzn (Birds Eye)	3.3 oz	20	none
Spinach, cooked	½ cup	21	none
Spinach, Creamed, frzn (Birds Eye)	3 oz	60	none
Spinach, raw	3½ oz	26	none
Spinach souffle (Home recipe)	1 cup	218	184
Spinach & Water Chestnuts, frzn (Birds Eye)	½ cup	29	none
Squash, Cooked Winter, frzn (Birds Eye)	4 oz	45	none
Swiss chard	½ cup	3	none
Vegetables & Rice, French Style, *International,* frzn (Birds Eye)	3.3 oz	110	none
Vegetables & Rice, Italian Style, *International,* frzn (Birds Eye)	3.3 oz	120	none
Vegetables & Rice, Spanish Style, *International,* frzn (Birds Eye)	3.3 oz	110	none

WAFFLES
(*see also* CREPES, FRENCH TOAST, PANCAKES/HOT CAKES)

FOOD	PORTION SIZE	CALORIES	CHOLESTEROL (Mg)
Waffle (Home recipe)	7"	282	70
Waffle (Home recipe)	9"	602	150

WENDY'S

FOOD	PORTION SIZE	CALORIES	CHOLESTEROL (Mg)
Bacon Cheeseburger, White Bun	1	460	65
Breakfast Sandwich	1	370	200
Chicken Fried Steak	1	580	95

FOOD	PORTION SIZE	CALORIES	CHOLESTEROL (Mg)
Chicken Sandwich, Multigrain Bun	1	320	59
Chili	8 oz	260	30
Double Hamburger, White Bun	1	560	125
Fish Fillet	1	210	45
French Fries, reg	1	280	15
French Toast	2	400	115
Frosty Dairy Dessert	1	400	50
Home Fries	1	360	20
Hot Stuffed Baked Potatoes, Bacon & Cheese	1	570	22
Hot Stuffed Baked Potatoes, Broccoli & Cheese	1	500	22
Hot Stuffed Baked Potatoes, Cheese	1	590	22
Hot Stuffed Baked Potatoes, Chili & Cheese	1	510	22
Hot Stuffed Baked Potatoes, Plain	1	250	tr
Hot Stuffed Baked Potatoes, Sour Cream & Chives	1	460	15
Kid's Meal Hamburger, 2 oz	1	220	20
Omelet, Ham & Cheese	1	250	450
Omelet, Ham, Cheese, Mushroom	1	290	355
Omelet, Ham, Cheese, Onion & Green Pepper	1	280	525
Omelet, Mushroom, Onion & Green Pepper	1	210	460
Single Hamburger, Multigrain Bun	1	340	67
Single Hamburger, White Bun	1	350	65
Taco Salad	1	390	40

FOOD	PORTION SIZE	CALORIES	CHOLESTEROL (Mg)

WHATABURGER

FOOD	PORTION SIZE	CALORIES	CHOLESTEROL (Mg)
Apple pie	1	236	1
Breakfast On A Bun	1	520	234
Egg Omelet Sandwich	1	312	191
French Fries, lg	1	332	1
French Fries, reg	1	221	1
Justaburger	1	265	25
Justaburger w/Cheese	1	312	37
Onion Rings	1	226	1
Pancakes w/o Syrup & Butter	1	199	34
Pancakes & Sausage w/o Syrup & Butter	1	407	77
Pecan Danish	1	270	12
Sausage	1	208	43
Taquito	1	310	223
Taquito w/Cheese	1	357	235
Vanilla Shake, extra lg	1	861	98
Vanilla Shake, lg	1	647	74
Vanilla Shake, med	1	433	49
Vanilla Shake, sm	1	322	37
Whataburger	1	580	70
Whataburger w/Cheese	1	669	96
Whataburger Double Meat	1	806	154
Whataburger Double Meat w/ Cheese	1	895	180
Whataburger Jr.	1	304	30
Whataburger Jr. w/Cheese	1	351	42
Whatacatch	1	475	34
Whatacatch w/Cheese	1	522	45
Whatachick'n Sandwich	1	671	71

WHEAT GERM

FOOD	PORTION SIZE	CALORIES	CHOLESTEROL (Mg)
WHEAT GERM	¼ cup	107	none

FOOD	PORTION SIZE	CALORIES	CHOLESTEROL (Mg)
WHIPPED TOPPINGS (*see also* CREAM)			
Cool Whip, Extra Creamy, frzn (Birds Eye)	1 Tbsp	16	none
Cool Whip, Non-Dairy, frzn (Birds Eye)	1 Tbsp	12	none
D-Zerta *Reduced Calorie Whipped Topping* Mix (General Foods)	1 Tbsp	8	none
Dream Whip Mix; as prep w/ whole milk (General Foods)	1 Tbsp	10	none
La Creme (Kraft)	1 Tbsp	12	none
Pressurized (Generic)	1 Tbsp	11	none
Real Cream Topping (Kraft)	¼ cup	25	10
Whip N' Top Mix	1 Tbsp	3	none
Whipped cream	1 Tbsp	8	2
Whipped Topping (Kraft)	¼ cup	35	none
Whipped Topping, frzn (Dover Farms)	1 Tbsp	17	1
Whipped topping, frzn (Generic)	1 Tbsp	13	none
Whipped topping mix, dry; prep w/whole milk (Generic)	1 Tbsp	8	tr
WINE (*see also* BEER, LIQUOR/LIQUEURS)			
Champagne	4 oz	84	none
Muscatel	3½ oz	158	none
Red wine	3½ oz	76	none
Rose	3½ oz	72	none
Sauterne	3½ oz	84	none
Sherry	2 oz	84	none
Vermouth, dry	3½ oz	105	none

FOOD	PORTION SIZE	CALORIES	CHOLESTEROL (Mg)
Vermouth, sweet	3½ oz	167	none
White wine	3½ oz	80	none

YOGURT

(*see also* YOGURT, FROZEN; YOGURT SHAKE)

There are regional differences in the fat content of *Yoplait* Yogurts. Those made in and/or distributed from California have higher fat and calorie content.

FOOD	PORTION SIZE	CALORIES	CHOLESTEROL (Mg)
All Varieties (Dannon)	8 oz	200	10
All Varieties, *Extra Smooth* (Dannon)	6 oz	190	10
All Varieties, *Extra Smooth Mini-Pack* (Dannon)	4.4 oz	130	10
All Varieties, Flavored, Whole Milk (Columbo)	3½ oz	93	9
All Varieties, *Original Mini-Pack* (Dannon)	4.4 oz	130	5
Apple Cinnamon, *Breakfast Style Yoplait* (General Mills)	6 oz	200	<10
Banana Custard Style, *Yoplait* (General Mills)	6 oz	190	10
Berries, *Breakfast Style, Yoplait* (General Mills)	6 oz	230	<10
Blueberry *Custard Style, Yoplait* (General Mills)	6 oz	190	10 to 25
Cherry w/Almonds, *Breakfast Style, Yoplait* (General Mills)	6 oz	210	<10
Coffee, lowfat (Generic)	8 oz	193	11
Coffee, lowfat, 1.5% fat (Friendship)	8 oz	210	14
Fruit, lowfat (Generic)	8 oz	232	9
Fruit, Lowfat, 1.5% fat (Friendship)	8 oz	230	14

FOOD	PORTION SIZE	CALORIES	CHOLESTEROL (Mg)
Fruit Flavors, *Original Style Yoplait* (General Mills)	6 oz	190	10 to 25
Fruit, *Hearty Nuts & Raisins* (Dannon)	8 oz	260	10
Fruit-On-The-Bottom (Dannon)	8 oz	240	10
Fruit On The Bottom Nonfat Lite, (Columbo)	3½ oz	88	none
Fruit On The Bottom, Whole Milk (Columbo)	3½ oz	110	9
Fruit, Mixed Berry *Custard Style, Yoplait* (General Mills)	6 oz	180	10 to 25
Fruit, *Supreme* (Dannon)	6 oz	190	15
Fruits, Citrus, *Breakfast Style, Yoplait* (General Mills)	6 oz	250	<10
Fruits, Orchard, *Breakfast Style, Yoplait* (General Mills)	6 oz	230	<10
Fruits, Tropical, *Breakfast Style, Yoplait* (General Mills)	6 oz	230	<10
Lemon *Custard Style, Yoplait* (General Mills)	6 oz	190	10 to 25
Peach, Sunrise, *Breakfast Style, Yoplait* (General Mills)	6 oz	230	<10
Plain (Dannon)	8 oz	140	10
Plain, lowfat (Generic)	1 oz (2 Tbsp)	18	2
Plain, lowfat (Generic)	8 oz	143	14
Plain, *Nonfat Lite* (Columbo)	8 oz	110	tr
Plain, *Original Style Yoplait* (General Mills)	6 oz	130	20 to 25
Plain, skim milk (Generic)	8 oz	127	5
Plain, 3.5% fat (Friendship)	8 oz	170	30
Plain, Whole Milk (Columbo)	3½ oz	66	9
Plain, Whole milk (Generic)	8 oz	138	30
Plain, yogurt cheese (Home recipe)	1 oz	20	7

FOOD	PORTION SIZE	CALORIES	CHOLESTEROL (Mg)
Raspberry *Custard Style*, *Yoplait* (General Mills)	6 oz	190	10 to 25
Strawberry, *Light N' Lively* (Kraft)	8 oz	160	10
Strawberry *Custard Style*, *Yoplait* (General Mills)	6 oz	190	10 to 25
Strawberry w/Almonds, *Breakfast Style*, *Yoplait* (General Mills)	6 oz	210	<10
Strawberry-Banana, *Breakfast Style*, *Yoplait* (General Mills)	6 oz	240	<10
Vanilla *Custard Style*, *Yoplait* (General Mills)	6 oz	180	10 to 25
Vanilla, lowfat (Generic)	8 oz	193	11
Vanilla, Lowfat, 1.5% fat (Friendship)	8 oz	210	14
Vanilla, *Nonfat Lite* (Columbo)	8 oz	160	tr

YOGURT, FROZEN
(*see also* ICE CREAM & FROZEN DESERTS)

FOOD	PORTION SIZE	CALORIES	CHOLESTEROL (Mg)
Danny On A Stick (Dannon)	1 bar	65	5
Danny On A Stick, Chocolate/Carob Coated (Dannon)	1 bar	135	5
Danny-Yo (Dannon)	½ cup	110	5
Raspberry (Sealtest)	4 oz	100	5
Soft Banana (Yoplait)	3 oz	90	15
Sorbet Swirl (Columbo)	4 oz	99	none
Tofree (Columbo)	4 oz	130	none
Vanilla (Columbo)	4 oz	102	7

FOOD	PORTION SIZE	CALORIES	CHOLESTEROL (Mg)

YOGURT SHAKE
(*see also* YOGURT; YOGURT, FROZEN)

FOOD	PORTION SIZE	CALORIES	CHOLESTEROL (Mg)
Cherry, *To-Fittness Instant Goody Two Shakes;* as prep w/2% milk	.67 oz pkg	140	15
Cherry, *To-Fittness Instant Goody Two Shakes;* as prep w/whole milk	.67 oz pkg	160	25
Raspberry, *To-Fittness Instant Goody Two Shakes;* as prep w/2% milk	.67 oz pkg	140	15
Raspberry, *To-Fittness Instant Goody Two Shakes;* as prep w/whole milk	.67 oz pkg	160	25

YORKSHIRE PUDDING
(*see* BREAD & ROLLS)

ZANTIGO

FOOD	PORTION SIZE	CALORIES	CHOLESTEROL (Mg)
Beef Enchilada	1	315	49
Cheese Enchilada	1	390	63
Hot Chilito	1	329	32
Mild Chilito	1	330	26
Taco	1	198	31
Taco Burrito	1	415	44

APPENDIX

Cholesterol Values of Selected Baby Foods

Strained foods packed for infant feeding are often used to feed adults when they cannot chew regular foods. It is for this reason that we include the following products. It is neither necessary nor desirable to limit cholesterol intake in infant and toddler diets.

FOOD	PORTION SIZE	CALORIES	CHOLESTEROL (Mg)
STRAINED MEAT			
Beef (Gerber)	1 jar (3½ oz)	96	29
Chicken (Gerber)	1 jar (3½ oz)	138	61
Ham (Gerber)	1 jar (3½ oz)	111	24
Lamb (Gerber)	1 jar (3½ oz)	101	38
Pork (Gerber)	1 jar (3½ oz)	107	35
Turkey (Gerber)	1 jar (3½ oz)	135	59
Veal (Gerber)	1 jar (3½ oz)	99	26
Egg yolks (Gerber)	1 jar (3½ oz)	198	622

FOOD	PORTION SIZE	CALORIES	CHOLESTEROL (Mg)

JUNIOR MEAT

FOOD	PORTION SIZE	CALORIES	CHOLESTEROL (Mg)
Beef (Gerber)	1 jar (3½ oz)	104	27
Chicken (Gerber)	1 jar (3½ oz)	145	59
Chicken Sticks (Gerber)	1 jar (2½ oz)	110	65
Ham (Gerber)	1 jar (3½ oz)	120	29
Lamb (Gerber)	1 jar (3½ oz)	102	41
Meat Sticks (Gerber)	1 jar (2½ oz)	110	33
Turkey (Gerber)	1 jar (3½ oz)	135	53
Turkey Sticks (Gerber)	1 jar (2½ oz)	120	61
Veal (Gerber)	1 jar (3½ oz)	102	27

STRAINED HIGH MEAT DINNERS

FOOD	PORTION SIZE	CALORIES	CHOLESTEROL (Mg)
Beef w/Vegetables (Gerber)	1 jar (4½ oz)	120	14
Chicken w/Vegetables (Gerber)	1 jar (4½ oz)	140	21
Ham w/Vegetables (Gerber)	1 jar (4½ oz)	100	12
Turkey w/Vegetables (Gerber)	1 jar (4½ oz)	130	19
Veal w/Vegetables (Gerber)	1 jar (4½ oz)	100	12

FOOD	PORTION SIZE	CALORIES	CHOLESTEROL (Mg)

JUNIOR HIGH MEAT DINNERS

FOOD	PORTION SIZE	CALORIES	CHOLESTEROL (Mg)
Beef w/Vegetables (Gerber)	1 jar (4½ oz)	130	15
Chicken w/Vegetables (Gerber)	1 jar (4½ oz)	130	26
Ham w/Vegetables (Gerber)	1 jar (4½ oz)	110	14
Turkey w/Vegetables (Gerber)	1 jar (4½ oz)	140	20
Veal w/Vegetables (Gerber)	1 jar (4½ oz)	110	12

STRAINED DINNERS

FOOD	PORTION SIZE	CALORIES	CHOLESTEROL (Mg)
Beef Egg Noodle (Gerber)	1 jar (4½ oz)	90	6
Cereal Egg Yolk w/Bacon (Gerber)	1 jar (4½ oz)	100	64
Chicken Noodle (Gerber)	1 jar (4½ oz)	80	10
Cream of Chicken Soup (Gerber)	1 jar (4½ oz)	70	12
Macaroni Cheese (Gerber)	1 jar (4½ oz)	90	3
Macaroni Tomato Beef (Gerber)	1 jar (4½ oz)	80	3
Turkey Rice (Gerber)	1 jar (4½ oz)	80	15
Vegetables Bacon (Gerber)	1 jar (4½ oz)	100	4
Vegetable Beef (Gerber)	1 jar (4½ oz)	80	5
Vegetable Chicken (Gerber)	1 jar (4½ oz)	80	7

FOOD	PORTION SIZE	CALORIES	CHOLESTEROL (Mg)
Vegetables Ham (Gerber)	1 jar (4½ oz)	80	4
Vegetable Lamb (Gerber)	1 jar (4½ oz)	90	3
Vegetable Turkey (Gerber)	1 jar (4½ oz)	70	12

JUNIOR DINNERS

FOOD	PORTION SIZE	CALORIES	CHOLESTEROL (Mg)
Beef Egg Noodle (Gerber)	1 jar (7½ oz)	140	12
Chicken Noodle (Gerber)	1 jar (7½ oz)	120	18
Macaroni Tomato Beef (Gerber)	1 jar (7½ oz)	130	4
Spaghetti Tomato Sauce Beef (Gerber)	1 jar (7½ oz)	140	9
Split Peas Ham (Gerber)	1 jar (7½ oz)	150	5
Turkey Rice (Gerber)	1 jar (7½ oz)	120	24
Vegetable Bacon (Gerber)	1 jar (7½ oz)	180	7
Vegetable Beef (Gerber)	1 jar (7½ oz)	140	9
Vegetable Chicken (Gerber)	1 jar (7½ oz)	120	17
Vegetable Ham (Gerber)	1 jar (7½ oz)	140	9
Vegetable Lamb (Gerber)	1 jar (7½ oz)	140	6
Vegetable Turkey (Gerber)	1 jar (7½ oz)	120	24

FOOD	PORTION SIZE	CALORIES	CHOLESTEROL (Mg)

CHUNKY FOODS

FOOD	PORTION SIZE	CALORIES	CHOLESTEROL (Mg)
Beef & Egg Noodles w/ Vegetables (Gerber)	1 jar (6 oz)	130	13
Potatoes & Ham (Gerber)	1 jar (6 oz)	110	7
Spaghetti, Tomato Sauce & Beef (Gerber)	1 jar (6.25 oz)	130	10
Vegetables & Beef (Gerber)	1 jar (6.25 oz)	120	10
Vegetables & Chicken (Gerber)	1 jar (6.25 oz)	120	16
Vegetables & Ham (Gerber)	1 jar (6.25 oz)	120	10
Vegetables & Turkey (Gerber)	1 jar (6.25 oz)	110	20

BAKED GOODS

FOOD	PORTION SIZE	CALORIES	CHOLESTEROL (Mg)
Arrowroot Cookies (Gerber)	2 cookies	50	<1
Toddler Biter Biscuits (Gerber)	1 piece	50	<1
Animal Crackers (Gerber)	4 crackers	50	<1
Pretzels (Gerber)	2 pieces	50	none
Zwieback Toast (Gerber)	2 pieces	60	<1

STRAINED DESSERTS

FOOD	PORTION SIZE	CALORIES	CHOLESTEROL (Mg)
Banana Apple (Gerber)	1 jar (4½ oz)	100	none
Cherry Vanilla Pudding (Gerber)	1 jar (4½ oz)	90	3
Chocolate Custard Pudding (Gerber)	1 jar (4½ oz)	90	14
Dutch Apple (Gerber)	1 jar (4½ oz)	100	4

FOOD	PORTION SIZE	CALORIES	CHOLESTEROL (Mg)
Fruit Dessert (Gerber)	1 jar (4½ oz)	100	none
Hawaiian Delight (Gerber)	1 jar (4½ oz)	120	2
Orange Pudding (Gerber)	1 jar (4½ oz)	110	11
Peach Cobbler (Gerber)	1 jar (4½ oz)	100	none
Vanilla Custard Pudding (Gerber)	1 jar (4½ oz)	110	15

JUNIOR DESSERTS

Banana Apple (Gerber)	1 jar (7½ oz)	150	none
Cherry Vanilla Pudding (Gerber)	1 jar (7½ oz)	160	7
Dutch Apple (Gerber)	1 jar (7½ oz)	160	9
Fruit Desert (Gerber)	1 jar (7½ oz)	160	none
Hawaiian Delight (Gerber)	1 jar (7½ oz)	190	3
Peach Cobbler (Gerber)	1 jar (7½ oz)	160	none
Vanilla Custard Pudding (Gerber)	1 jar (7½ oz)	190	29